"If you always put limits in everything you do, physical or anything else, it will spread into your work and into your life. There are no limits. There are only plateaus, and you must not stay there. You must *go beyond* them."

-*Bruce Lee*

The Monk Life
& Central Power

HAIDER ALI ELAHI-KHAN

CONTENTS

INTRODUCTION

This book is designed to benefit readers in a variety of ways, increasing their health & fitness, through physical, mental & nutritional fortitude, and to then begin developing 'Central Power'.

Central Power is the structural anatomy of human inner force, advanced breathing techniques and muscular movements originating from Bromo Mountain in Indonesia, an active Volcano.

The book is divided into four chapters, discussing each element of 'fortitude' based on the writer's knowledge gained through his background in boxing and Indonesian Martial Arts – ancient techniques that lay the foundation for 'Kei', otherwise known as 'Chi', 'Central Power' or 'Inner Strength'.

The book is designed to benefit everyone, whether you are a beginner, a professional athlete, trainer, coach, regular gym-goer, into health & nutrition, sick and gravely ill, frail or elderly, disabled, over thirty or forty years old and looking for a new dimension to achieve great and long-lasting health into old age.

Of course if you are a professional coach, athlete or nutritionist, you may find the last three chapters contain information that you already know, perhaps even more so than the author. However, these chapters are here so that *anyone* can pick up the book and find a total solution, physically, mentally and nutritionally that help generate 'Central Power' because ultimately, the first chapter – 'Central Power', requires the use of mental, physical and nutritional fortitude to achieve the best results. The first chapter, is where *professionals* in sport would find the most benefit, however they may like to see which techniques and nutrition the author found to be of the best fit. Furthermore, mental health issues, nutritional imbalance, affects us all.

The term, The Monk Life, originates from the author's description of his clean-living lifestyle. The author comes from a background in boxing, albeit not professional, but the lifestyle of training, nutrition, mental strength and *Central Power* provided the perfect recipe for optimum health. Monks, live a life of seclusion, practicing their arts, strengthening their mind, body and soul to achieve optimum results. Elements of this lifestyle are beneficial to us as we get older, or train for a purpose. For example, Rocky Marciano, the professional boxer who retired undefeated, when training for a fight was like a Monk - he secluded himself from his family, sometimes for up to three months before a fight, he watched his diet, weight and muscle tone. A week before a fight he would avoid mail, phone calls and meeting people. He would not even shake hands (to avoid getting sick) or go for a car ride, or try any new foods. Other boxers, people in the fight-game, go through similar life-changes when training. These types of changes, are ideal to increase fortitude in the areas defined in this book, and ultimately provide a foundation to start the techniques of Central Power – which in turn, give *you*, the foundation to achieve 'Kei" or 'Chi', or as the author defines it, 'Inner Fortitude'.

The author, is a master of 'Kei', having trained for over a decade in Indonesia, and the purpose of writing this book is *not* to boast or brag, nor to undermine the great work professionals in the field of sports science and coaching do, but to serve them and the general public through his knowledge. This book teaches the foundation 'breathing techniques' and the 'muscle-lock' movements, as a starting point to aid the reader in achieving the best possible health he or she can.

Additionally, the author is aware that each person represents their own physiology – what works for them, may or *may not* work for another. However, the author advises to take what you can from the book, see what works for you. The first chapter will benefit everyone – as long as you can *concentrate*.

The benefits in the last three chapters are numerous in themselves, following a life of healthy eating, living and training pays dividends to the state of your internal organs, blood vessels, blood flow and mental strength - weaknesses can diminish but in some cases this requires intense work and therapy. Once this is combined with the foundations of 'Inner Fortitude', the benefits start to become immense. These include, but are not limited to: focus, increased physical strength, endurance, confidence, increased ability to take a punch, strengthened interior-muscles particularly around the internal organs, improved posture, a strengthened core, abdominal area and the beginning of Central Power delivery.

The knowledge contained here on the foundations of Kei, is approximately 10% of the authors complete knowledge of the subject, however it will benefit everyone – from athletes to the elderly, children, disabled people, sick and gravely ill people who cannot exercise – as long as they can still focus & *breathe*.

People have used these ancient techniques for millennia, developing them into Kei, and thus enabling them to perform formidable athletic acts, as well as acting as a form of healing therapy for the sick. The author himself, was well known for power-punching an Iron plate *fourteen times in four seconds* without suffering *pain or injury*, a video still available on YouTube. As well as *three-finger press-ups on one hand*. In his fighting days, he called himself the 'Hands of Stone' after the great Roberto Duran. However, these days he is more of a boxing fan, businessman and author. As with most challenges in life, another benefit of Central Power, the better you get at it and the more you practice, the more results you will see over time.

The author would be pleased to learn of anyone who has benefitted from the book, and if there are any questions feel free to contact the author on his social media (located at the back of the book). The author has boxed and fought in boxing gyms across the U.K and Indonesia, and understands the pains boxers go through to achieve results, thus it would be rewarding for the author to learn if fighters have benefitted from this book.

The author wishes the best for everyone who reads this book, hopefully, it will serve you well.

CENTRAL POWER & INNER FORTITUDE

'I am learning to understand, rather than immediately judge
or be judged. I cannot blindly follow the crowd and except
their approach. I will not allow myself to indulge in the
usual manipulating game of role creation. Fortunately for
me, my self-knowledge has transcended that I have come to
understand that life is best to be lived and not
conceptualized. I am happy because I am growing daily and I
am honestly not knowing where the limit lies. To be certain,
every day there can be a *new* revelation or discovery. I
treasure the memory of the past misfortunes, it has added
more to my bank of *fortitude*.'
-*Bruce Lee*

The bank of *fortitude*. This is what The Monk Life intends to
provide for you, to fill your bank of fortitude, to give you a
new revelation and discovery that can potentially change
your life, forever, and for the better. To give you long lasting
health and help you, overcome *your* life challenges.

The following chapters discuss the importance of physical
health and how to achieve it, the importance of mental
health and ways to alleviate it, the importance of nutritional
intake and how to improve it, all in order to put us in the
optimal condition for Central Power delivery: the
foundations of Kei, inner strength, and inner fortitude.
However, to achieve optimal condition takes time, and not
all of us are in or ever will be in a position to get there.
Therefore you may practice these foundation techniques
regardless of your condition. As long you can focus, breathe,
make certain subtle 'lock' movements, you will succeed. If
you are gravely ill, you can practice as you lay down, if you

are disabled you can adjust, if you are mentally unwell, learn to focus your 'pupils', if you are elderly, you can *still* achieve Central Power. No one, is off limits.

The key, is to learn to 'focus the pupils'. Without focusing the pupils, you will be unable to develop Central Power through these techniques. We will discuss methods of how to do this later.

Central Power is an ancient technique that gives the mind and body greater control over the central nervous system and internal muscles. The benefits are numerous, increasing awareness, confidence, instincts, inner strength, greater strength and ability to withstand punishment, power, focus, balance, core strength, strengthening of the muscles around the internal organs, improved heart rate, lowers blood pressure, improves overall health and wellbeing, posture, blood flow and so on. It can be applied to any activity we undertake, it can be practiced under any circumstances, it is *you*, in control of your focus, your breathing, your internal muscles. For a fighter, it can improve your endurance, engine and ability to withstand punishment.

This is done by stimulating the right and left hemispheres of the brain through the pupils, which in turn alternates simultaneously down your spine, crossing over through the central nervous system and into the 'muscular system' or internal muscles – the first muscles we use for this, are the lower stomach muscles. Try it now, tense your lower stomach muscles, keep it there, relax every other part of your body, but keep your lower stomach muscles tensed, or 'pulled in', the level of force, for now, is up to you. Just practice the art of keeping it tense, and take a long breath in, hold it, and take a long breath out, breathing only through your nose, keeping your stomach 'in' and 'tensed' throughout each breath.

The spinal cord is attached to the part of the brain called the brainstem and runs through the spinal canal. Cranial nerves exit the brainstem, and nerve roots exit the spinal cord to both sides of the body. The spinal cord carries signals (messages) between the brain and the peripheral nerves. The central nervous system, controls most functions of the body and mind. This is how Central Power is created, strengthened and delivered to the parts of the body that we want it to. Ancient breathing techniques, and an 'interior muscle-lock' system are what stimulate the brain, to send messages through the central nervous system and the spinal cord, to start generating Central Power. Imagine starting a car but now you can start tuning the engine to deliver more torque, more power, acceleration, etc. The process involves using the pupils, the brain, the CNS, the interior/exterior muscular system and other organs (such as your lungs) *simultaneously*, in order for Central Power to begin generation.

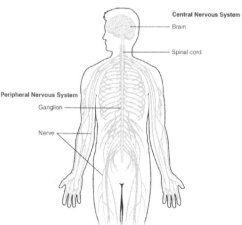

Source: Wikipedia

Stimulation only occurs when the pupils are focused in '*one direction*'. They cannot move during the exercises. Try it now, focus on something, hold your pupils, keep your lower stomach muscles tensed, and breathe in till your lungs are full, count to ten, then exhale, maintaining the mentioned conditions until your lungs are empty, then relax.

The 'one-lock' system combines the breathing techniques with subtle body movements that lock each muscle in place. In this chapter you will learn the first three locks. The muscular system is responsible for the movement of the human body. Attached to the bones of the skeletal system are about seven hundred named muscles that make up roughly half of a person's body weight. Each of these muscles is a discrete organ constructed of skeletal muscle tissue, blood vessels, tendons, and nerves. Muscle tissue is also found inside of the heart, digestive organs, and blood vessels. Central Power attempts to use the muscular system to deliver 'Kei', via the route described.

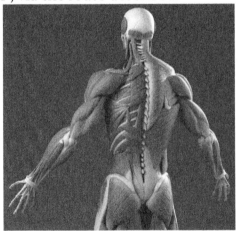

Source: GraphicVizion

Numerous scientific studies are starting to show how controlled breathing can positively affect mental *and* physical health. A 2016 study stumbled upon the neural circuit in the brainstem, that plays a key-role in the breathing-brain connection. Research suggests that *slowing* your breathing increases "baroreflex sensitivity," the mechanism that regulates blood pressure via heart rate. Over time, using controlled breathing to lower blood pressure and heart rate may lower risk of stroke and cerebral aneurysm, and generally *decreases stress* on blood vessels (a big plus for cardiovascular health).

A recent study showed that controlling breathing by counting breaths influences 'neuronal oscillations throughout the brain', particularly in brain regions related to emotion. Brain activity (monitored by EEG) in regions related to emotion, memory and *awareness* showed a more organized pattern versus what is normally experienced during a resting state. The results are preliminary, but add to the argument that controlling breathing taps into a deeper level of control and power.

A 2016 study showed for the first time that the rhythm of our breathing generates electrical activity in the brain which in turn influences how well we remember. The biggest differences were linked to whether the study participants were inhaling or exhaling, and whether they breathed through the *nose* or mouth. Researchers think that *nasal* inhalation triggers *greater electrical activity* in the amygdala, the brain's emotional epicenter, which enhances recall of fearful stimuli. Inhaling also seems linked to greater activity in the hippocampus, the seat of memory.

A recent study has suggested that controlled breathing may boost the immune system and improve energy metabolism. Whilst this is the most speculative of the study findings on this list, it is also one of the most *exciting*. The study was evaluating the 'Relaxation Response' (a term popularized in the 1970s book of the same name by Dr Herbert Benson, also a co-author of this study), which refers to a method of engaging the parasympathetic nervous system to counteract the nervous system's 'fight or flight' response to stress. Controlled breathing triggers a parasympathetic response, according to the theory, and may also improve resilience of the immune system. The study also found improvements in energy metabolism and more efficient insulin secretion, which results in better blood sugar management. The results support the conclusion that controlled breathing is not only a counterbalance to stress, but also valuable for improving overall health.

The above provides more evidence to suggest that what you are about to learn, will aid you in turning your life around, as it did for me all those years ago.

It was 2003 in Indonesia when I first met my teacher. A group of friends in one of my social circles practiced the art and introduced me. I remember the day clearly, we met up at one of our friends large houses. My teacher came with a bunch of other guys, who all became my good friends and instructors. I had no idea what we were going to do but I felt that it was is definitely for me, judging by the atmosphere around us. My training in fighting had long left me by then, I was in my early twenties and years of neglect and sedentary lifestyle had caused me to become overweight, lose agility, lose focus, motivation. Looking back, I was close to being finished, over the hill as they say. There was no way I could have fought again. But the one thing I did have that never leaves a true fighter, was the competitive spirit, the will and the self-belief. Muhammad Ali, the greatest boxer of all time, said 'the will, *must* be stronger than the skill', food for thought.

We sat down in a slightly darkened room, with a candle in front of us for focus. As our teacher guided us through the breathing exercises - I participated well. We also completed various physical fitness exercises, combining them to the breathing techniques. Then I saw the others perform 'Kei'. It was the most mesmerizing thing I had seen. What you will learn here, is the *foundation* of Kei: the foundation breathing techniques, the physical exercises and the first stages of the 'one-lock system'. In China, they call it Chi, in Indonesia and Japan, it is Kei. Our form of Kei, creates a high pitch sound (*a la* Bruce Lee) when performing the advanced breathing techniques, twenty five reps of which are equivalent to an hour of lifting weights without the unwanted side effects. Which is why I rarely lift weights unless it's deadlift, squat etc. as mentioned in chapter one. If you want to see Bruce Lee perform Kei, search on YouTube for the 'Fist of Fury', 'dojo fight scene', where Bruce Lee walks in with a sign, offensive to Chinese, he breaks it in half and proceeds towards the Japanese Master who ushers his students to attack him. He attacks the first two, then the students encircle him, at this point Bruce Lee goes into position, before he commits to his first attack on the group surrounding him, he performs 'Kei'.

Once our training session was over, around ninety minutes later, I could feel the difference in my solar plexus, my abdomen and my posture. Focusing on a flame with these techniques increases your focus substantially, so that had made a difference for me too. I was hooked.

I hung out with my teacher daily, he lived in the shanty towns of Jakarta, in Bidara Cina, Cawang. Brother Ote, shorted for *'oteda'* which stood for 'oleh raga, tenega dalam', which means *'the art of Central Power'*, and was also the basis of my nickname at the time, Ali Oteda.

We would hang out and train, day to day, I would go home and train again, practicing the lock systems, over and over.

Eventually, within six months to a year, I had surpassed those around me and developed Kei. Over the years we visited waterfalls in the mountains, some of the most beautiful places I have seen. We would sit at the base of the waterfall, so the water would land on us and practice locking and Kei. I remember one of the first times my teacher was doing Kei under the waterfall. All I remember was that it felt like I could see the tiny droplets of water around him, like they had paused, giving an almost an electrical feeling for a few seconds. This was 2003. I would also like to mention here that I had seen my teacher over the years perform acts of *healing* using Kei directed into the solar plexus of another individual, causing them to rise from an unconscious state with a *smile* and clear eyes. I saw this twice, both times the unconscious state was from a drug overdose, a side effect of the poor shanty towns surrounding the rich urban areas of Jakarta.

I stood under the waterfall, which felt like rocks landing on you, however when you focus, and use the techniques, this only strengthens you, there is no pain, nor injury, only gain, when you 'lock'.

We trained together for years, until I finally returned to England. Whilst training, I had become a Master of Kei, utilizing higher, advanced ancient methods of breathing, locking, balancing, unbeknown to the average man, with documentary knowledge passed down to me from my master, with detailed instructions of how to perform each technique, using ancient knowledge from a secret book. When I returned to England I was reborn as an athlete and fighter, I was in better condition than I had been before I left. Although I didn't turn professional as a boxer, I trained with the best, including a welterweight British Champion. I boxed in different gyms across the U.K, I had many 'gym fights', a handful of amateur fights in the U.K and some fights in Indonesia. I gave up boxing, my 'Iron Punch Technique' was well known that at one point I trained with the U.S. Contenders from the famous reality TV show, becoming lifelong friends with their Coach, Nettles Nasser from the Bronx. I also created a lifelong friendship with the three time world champion, in two divisions, 'Sweet' Reggie Johnson, who fought Roy Jones Jnr, and who fought James Toney, a fight he arguably won. He also beat Steve Collins handily. I met Spencer 'The Knowledge' Fearon on my boxing journey, a great man and boxing pundit for Sky Sports, who provided great advice and friendship. As a hobby, I took up Close Protection as Military and Government personnel from Indonesia wanted me around them in London. To this day I have kept up my training to a similar level – but not quite as intense as a professional boxer. A professional boxer utilizes his regime twenty-four seven, trains hard, and cuts no corners, because this is his or hers livelihood, and they need to be on top form for the one-on-one fight in the ring. Being mentally strong in fights is the most important tool to have, exceeding your counterparts in lifestyle and training, with the slightest edge, can lead to victory.

I have not had professional fights, however I have been in the ring and boxed. If I mentioned *only* three fights, that describe the benefits of Central Power to you they would be because in the first two, the opponent saw me training and pulled out of the fight, defeating your opponent *mentally*, is your first task. For the third fight, they gave me the most cushioned, old gloves you could find whilst he wore new and thinner gloves. I still proceeded to outbox him comfortably. These techniques will not miraculously give you a good engine to go twelve rounds as professional boxers do, but they will improve a great deal on whatever engine you do have. From helping you to control your heart rate when it is exceedingly fast to substantially improving your ability to take a punch and withstand punishment.

Inevitably, Central Power is very advantageous, a person whose training regime is monk-like, will perform brilliantly under the circumstances due to their dedication and commitment. Such a person is an athlete. If the person was to learn and apply Central Power, I have no doubt they would improve in all areas. Bruce Lee was a master of Central Power & Kei. It is well known amongst our circle that my teachers, teachers-teacher, taught Bruce Lee in Hong Kong. I am of the belief, Manny 'Pacman' Pacquiao, one of the greatest boxers of this generation, practices some form of Central Power, hence his unique ability, and rise in weight maintaining power with some accusing him, wrongfully so, of using performance enhancing drugs. Our secret, is Central Power, we do not need, illegal supplements, as The Monk Life shows. Now, at my later age, I am still able to compete if I wanted to, but I focus more on my training, serving others, and helping you, to overcome *your* challenges.

Let's talk about focus, and the first breathing technique 'nafas dalam', which means 'a deep, relaxed breath'. *Focus*. The definition of focus is defined as 'to pay particular attention to a central point'. In Central Power, we call this 'one direction concentration'. This is one of the core exercises you must learn to do. The pupils of the eyes, one of the most complex organs of the body, are connected to the brain via the optic nerve.

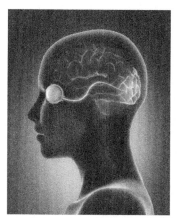

Source: Discovery Eye Foundation

Without the ability to focus, as I have mentioned earlier, you will be unable to develop Central Power. So how do we learn one direction-focus? Read on.

The only item we need to learn to focus on is a traditional *'candle'*. It is possible to use a dot on a piece of paper placed on a wall. However, the more traditional route is a candle; the candle flame is also easier to focus on. Some of the advanced breathing techniques that I know, involve multiple candles, so I would say that this is a *must* have requirement. Later, when you master these techniques you can use a dot on paper, because this helps when you are in situations where a candle is not available, for example at work.

Place the candle down in front of you. I prefer a slightly darkend room to enhance the candle flame. Light it, sit three feet away from the candle, crosslegged, on a firm surface like a yoga mat, hands resting on your knees, back straight, with your whole body relaxed, your lower stomach muscles are in the 'in' position, but without force, just gently. Now keep your eyes on the candle flame, blinking is okay. Practice focusing on the flame, for as long as you can. See Figure One.

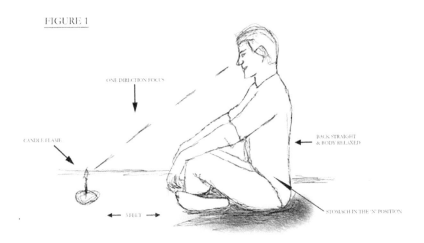

FIGURE 1

ONE DIRECTION FOCUS

CANDLE FLAME

BACK STRAIGHT
& BODY RELAXED

3 FEET

STOMACH IN THE 'IN' POSITION

Remember, eyes on the flame, stomach in the 'in' position, body relaxed, back straight, now empty all the air in your lungs through your nose. You will be inhaling and exhaling strictly through the nose for these exercises. Now, inhale through the nose, very slowly, a subtle breath-in, as you breathe in keep to the aforementioned conditions, your stomach should be pulled in further as you do.

Once your lungs are full, hold your breath for around ten seconds. If you cannot, try three and work your way up. Once you reach ten (or three), exhale the air through your nose, again, most importantly, keeping to the said conditions, stomach 'in', body relaxed, back straight, eyes 'focused' on the flame. Any interuption to your focus, will hinder your progress.

When the air in the lungs is empty, repeat the process. Aim for three times. Then five, then ten, as you improve. However, you can aim for three, then move on to the next breathing exercises, in sets of three, increasing each set as a whole. If you want to just practice this one consistently, you can do that too.

Try to aim for long, silent, subtle breaths, that last anything from ten seconds 'in', ten seconds 'hold', ten seconds 'out', then repeat – keeping the focus and conditions.
This is called 'nafas dalam', and is designed to help you relax, learn to focus and begin stimulating your organs for Central Power.
Refer to Figure One and let's review the conditions:
1. Eyes focused in one direction on the flame
2. Stomach in the 'in' position *at all times* throughout each breath
3. Body relaxed and back straight
4. Long, subtle breaths in and out through the nose, holding each breath from three upto ten seconds. Concentrate on the flame and your lower stomach muscles. If you can do fifteen, twenty etc., go for it, making sure the breaths 'in' and 'out' are just as long, and inhale, exhale all of the air in your lungs.
5. Repeat sets of three, then up to five, then ten, as you improve.

Now let's talk about the second breathing technique, known as *'one release'*.
One release, is identical to 'nafas dalam', with one major difference. The lower stomach muscles, abdominal muscles, solar plexus must *all* be tensed. My teacher used to focus more on the solar plexus, to strengthen the core, so we will do the same here. In order to tense the solar plexus, as hard

as you can, you must tense the whole abdominal muscles too.

One release should be performed immediately after performing 'nafas dalam', with the same number of sets, and your inhale, hold, exhale lengths should be of the same length, if you can. If you can't due to the difficulty of tensing the solar plexus, then hold for less. You will get there in time.

So, you inhale, keeping your stomach 'in' and 'tensed' throughout, once you are in the 'hold' position, tense your solar plexus, and keep it tensed throughout the exercise. As you exhale, keep the solar plexus tensed, repeat the process, three, five, or ten times, as you are capable of. This technique is difficult, the intensity can cause you to feel dizzy, so do it while seated. When you improve, you can do it anywhere. If you feel dizzy, stop, do 'nafas dalam', and start again. Later, we will apply one release to some physical fitness exercises.

Have a look at Figure Two, and let's review the conditions for 'one release':

    1.   Eyes focused in one direction on the flame

    2.   Stomach in the 'in' and 'tensed' position throughout

    3.   Body relaxed and back straight

    4.   Long, subtle but *slightly* more intense breaths (due to the tensing of your abdominal area), then 'hold' (hold for three, five or ten seconds), tense the solar plexus on 'hold'. Keep the solar plexus tensed throughout the 'hold' and 'exhale'.

    5.   Repeat, sets of three, five or ten.

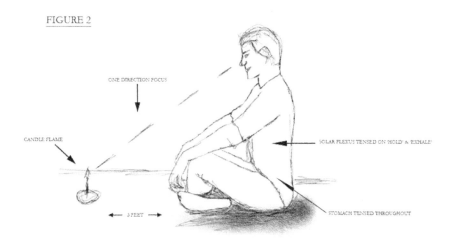

FIGURE 2

ONE DIRECTION FOCUS

SOLAR PLEXUS TENSED ON 'HOLD' & 'EXHALE'

CANDLE FLAME

STOMACH TENSED THROUGHOUT

← 3 FEET →

Now let's look at the third and final breathing exercise known as, 'three release'.

Three release is identical to one release, only that it differs in the way we exhale. With three release, we exhale in *three* stages, first 25% of your breath, followed by a 'hold', then another 25% of your breath, followed by another 'hold', then the last 50% of your breath is released.

So, in this third technique, we are keeping our stomach tensed, inhale, hold and tense the solar plexus, exhale 25%-hold-25%-hold-50%, keeping the solar plexus tensed throughout, then repeat. Each 'hold' can be three to five seconds long, or ten if you can. Three release should be performed immediately after one release. You can do 'nafas dalam' a few times in between each exercise, 'nafas dalam' should be your base technique, for cooling down and lowering your heart rate, in between sets.

Have a look at figure Three and let's review this technique:

1. Eyes focused in one direction on the flame
2. Stomach in the 'in' and 'tensed' position throughout
3. Body relaxed and back straight
4. Long, subtle but slightly more intense breaths (due to the tensing of the abdominal area), then 'hold' for three seconds (increase as you improve), tense the solar plexus on 'hold', and maintain this throughout
5. Exhale 25% of your breath, 'hold' again for three seconds
6. Exhale 25% of your breath, 'hold' again for three seconds
7. Exhale 50% of your breath
8. Repeat, sets of three, five, or ten as you improve

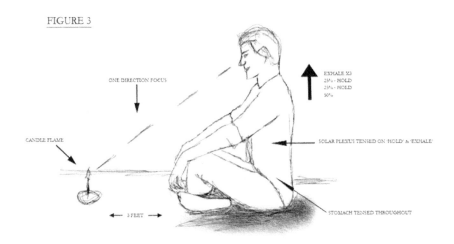

FIGURE 3

ONE DIRECTION FOCUS

CANDLE FLAME

3 FEET

EXHALE X3
25% - HOLD
25% - HOLD
50%

SOLAR PLEXUS TENSED ON 'HOLD' & 'EXHALE'

STOMACH TENSED THROUGHOUT

These techniques should be completed one after the other, it is possible to start with smaller sets of three, and stop. However, it would be better to apply a sixty minute session with physical fitness, as I will describe shortly. Each inhale and exhale should be long, through the nose, intense (for one release and three release). However, they shouldn't be done loudly, meaning be still, focus on your breath, the sound, if it is too loud, it is probably being done too fast. The keys to success are not breaking your one direction focus, inhaling, holding and exhaling with ease and for a good, equal length of time, tensing the solar plexus (for one and three release), keeping the stomach 'in' always (tensed for one and three release).

Once you complete this exercise, say for example a minimum set of three for each technique, lay down for two minutes, doing 'nafas dalam' as you lay down.

In order to enhance the above techniques, we must condition our muscles to endure more training, thus giving us the opportunity to progess further into Central Power. Strengthening the stomach muscles, solar plexus and chest help exploit the breathing techniques and enhance the muscular lock system. The start of the 'one-lock system' is where you want to be. To achieve this, follow these guidelines here for Central Power physical fitness.
As I mentioned earlier, one release will be the breathing technique you will use in each exercise. You will perform push-ups and sit ups, but not in the usual 'rep' form as you do in the gym, but imagine 'one release' applied to each 'rep'.

For example, imagine a traditional 'push up' (we prefer on the knuckles, but do as you are able to), when you are in the push up position, focus on the flame, before lowering, you inhale as you do in one release, hold and tense your solar plexus, at this point you lower yourself, hold for three seconds (or five, or ten) and exhale as you rise, keeping to the conditions. Count it as one set and repeat the exercise until you get to ten. Taking slow, deep breaths each time, with a tensed solar plexus in each 'hold' and 'exhale'. These exercises are adaptable and can be applied to many techniques in chapter one.

Once you improve, you can increase the number of push ups you do in one breath, i.e., when you 'hold', tense your solar plexus and lower yourself, instead of exhaling, complete three push ups, then exhale on the third. See if you can get to ten, ten reps of which would equal one hundred push ups in only ten breaths. But stick to one for now.

Let's review this technique, have a look at Figure Four:

1.   Eyes focused in one direction on the flame
2.   Go into push up position, and perform one release until 'hold' (breathing in, tensing the solar plexus and holding)
3.   On tensing the solar plexus, lower yourself
4.   'Hold' and then exhale whilst you rise, keeping to the conditons
5.   Repeat three, five, or ten times
6.   Try increasing the number of push ups you can complete in one breath, three, five, until you get to ten. In multiple push ups, there is no need to 'hold', just perform the push up.

FIGURE 4

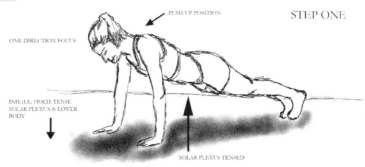

ONE DIRECTION FOCUS

PUSH-UP POSITION

STEP ONE

INHALE, HOLD, TENSE
SOLAR PLEXUS & LOWER
BODY

SOLAR PLEXUS TENSED

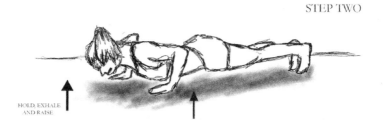

STEP TWO

HOLD, EXHALE
AND RAISE

TENSED

Now lets discuss the same technique, however this time it will be applied to the sit up.

Lay down flat with your arms beside your head (do not pull on the head), and your knees bent. This is known as the bent knee-sit up without restraints. This has been scientifically proven to strengthen the abdominals. Tests conducted by Dr Raymond Chong and his colleagues at the Medical College of Georgia concluded the traditional bent-knee sit up is a more thorough exercise than modern abdominal crunches and sit ups done using an exercise ball.

As you lay down flat, inhale as you would in one release. Focus on something around you, i.e. on the ceiling, as from this position it is difficult to focus on the flame without straining your neck, unless you place the flame on an elevated position. Tense the solar plexus, hold, and perform the sit up, once you reach your knees, hold for three seconds and exhale as you lower yourself. Repeat this ten times, and as before, when you improve you can increase to three, five and ten sit ups in each breath, culminating in one hundred sit ups in ten breaths.

Refer to Figure Five and let's review the exercise:

1. Eyes focused on a dot, or elevated flame
2. Get into bent knee-sit up position
3. Perform one release until 'hold'
4. On tensing the solar plexus, perform the sit up till you reach your knees or as far as you can go, and hold for three seconds
5. Exhale as you lower yourself, repeat, up to ten times
6. Try increasing the number of sit ups you can do in one breath, from three, five, to ten. Again, there is no need to 'hold' when performing multiple sit ups.

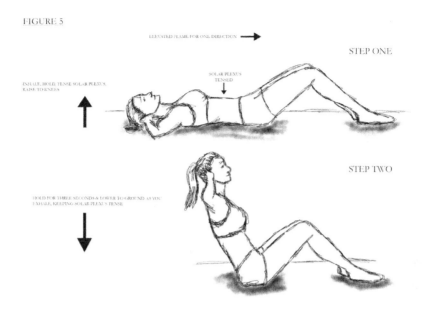

FIGURE 5

ELEVATED PLANE FOR ONE DIRECTION ➔

STEP ONE

SOLAR PLEXUS TENSED

INHALE, HOLD, TENSE SOLAR PLEXUS, RAISE TO KNEES

STEP TWO

HOLD FOR THREE SECONDS & LOWER TO GROUND AS YOU EXHALE, KEEPING SOLAR PLEXUS TENSE

Now let's discuss the final physical exercise you should apply before doing the foundations of the one-lock system. Please note, if you are unable to complete the physical exercises, due to being disabled, elderly, or ill, you may still train the breathing techniques and the lock system. The physical exercises are designed to enhance the system, you can also redesign the exercise to suit your needs. Such as a wheelchair bound person may do chin ups instead, and so on.

This exercise is known as 'the V position'. Lay down flat on the floor, on a firm surface such as a yoga mat. Keep your legs straight (or bent) and raise them forty-five degrees, keeping your toes pointed – if possible. Then, raise your body forty-five degrees (approximately), keeping your arms behind your head (*a la* sit up) or out in front of you for balance with your palms facing down, now you are in the 'V' position. Perform one release until 'hold'. Maintain the 'V' as you exhale, keeping your solar plexus tense throughout, perform one release consistently in the 'V' until you have to relax, perform 'nafas dalam', and repeat. Try it for upto three minutes, or five, as you are able to. Practice makes perfect. There is no failure in The Monk Life, once you commit to small, attainable goals, completed daily, you will achieve, it's just a matter of time.

Refer to Figure Six and let's review the conditons of this exercise:

1. Lay flat on your back
2. Raise your legs forty-five degrees (knees bent or straight), then your body forty-five degress to attain the 'V' position, arms out straight for balance, palms facing down, or behind your head (harder)
3. Eyes focused in one direction on the flame
4. Perform one release
5. Maintain 'V' and exhale, repeat one release in 'V' position
6. Perform as many one releases as you can, until you have to relax, perfrom 'nafas dalam' and try it again, for upto three, or five minutes

FIGURE 6

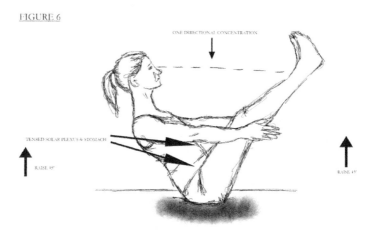

ONE DIRECTIONAL CONCENTRATION

TENSED SOLAR PLEXUS & STOMACH

RAISE 45°

RAISE 45°

We have now performed the three foundation breathing techniques, and three physical fitness exercises that compliment them. I would advise for you to keep trying, keep pushing yourself daily to achieve one or more of your small, attainable goals.

Failure, is nothing to fear. Bruce Lee said, 'Don't fear failure. Not failure, but low aim, is the crime. In great attempts it is glorious even to fail'. Heed the words. If you are taking minute steps towards your goal, from each chapter, you are *succeeding*. If you fail to complete a three mile jog, instead you completed a two mile brisk walk, you *succeeded*. The important thing is to keep trying, remain consistent. Remember The Monk Life philosophy, small, consistent changes, over the long term. This applies to your training, small, consistent sessions, over the long term. If you can make larger changes, then that's great, what's stopping you? *Nothing.* You are your only barrier to progress, for yourself, your family, if you don't take the steps to change your life now. If you have a disability, or illness, or you are elderly, dig deep, you will be surprised at what you are capable of.

There are many stories of elderly and disadvantaged people achieving new goals, look at the Paralympics, is something stopping them? They are *phenomenal* human beings. Find an inspiring person, learn from them.

When a newbie enters the boxing gym for the first time, he or she has no idea how to punch. The coach will teach them, they would try over and over again. Each time would either be worse or better than the first time. The person returns to the gym, week after week, eventually, that jab, that hook, that right hand is looking *exquisite*.

The same applies here, 'practice makes perfect'. If you fail in one push up, you still tried, if you fail in one sit up, you still tried, if it's taking you a while to get the gist of the breathing techniques, you *still* tried. Keep going, eventually you will get there. Adjust the physical exercises to suit your abilities and as long as you hold for a minimum of one count, that is a good start.

Muhammad Ali said, 'I hated every minute of training, but I said 'don't quit', suffer now and live the rest of your life as a champion'. You can be your *own* champion, *everyone*, has a champion within them. You have to find it.

He also said, 'The fight is won or lost far away from the witnesses – behind the lines, in the gym, and out there on the road, long before I dance under those lights'. He is referring to the training you have to do, the mental, physical, nutritional preparation you have to do in the confines of your own four walls, *before* you go out there and face the world as a stronger, more confident, healthier human being. It depends what you do, in your own time, that will improve *you*, and create a *new* you.

Now let's move on to the one-lock system. The one-lock system, as I mentioned earlier is the system that begins locking, or utilizing the 'muscular system'. It consists nine stages, this book, will teach you the first three.

Refer to Figure Seven. As you can see, you are sitting in the same position as you were for the breathing techniques. Cross legged, on a firm surface, hands on your knees, body relaxed, back straight, eyes focused in one direction on the flame.

What you are about to do is similar to one release, but with an additional 'lock', in a particular order, and then exhale. This will involve locking the stomach, and now the 'chest', and then the solar plexus, followed by 'hold', and then exhale. 'Three locks' in 'one breath'. In each movement you should feel each set of muscles lock into place, in the order described, stomach, chest and finally, the solar plexus. Locking the chest is a very subtle, circular movement. I will do my best to describe it, and display it in Figure Seven. Inhale as you would in one release, tightening the lower stomach muscles on 'hold', as hard as you can. Now you need to perform a 360 degrees movement involving the shoulders from the joints.

Your body is relaxed, imagine lifting your shoulders from the joints in a circular movement, that goes away from you ever-so-slightly, then in a circular motion upwards, then back towards you, then downwards, till it reaches behind you, down in a circular motion, as much as you can take it, back to the original starting point, and perhaps further 'in', a full 360 degrees, you should feel the chest lock into place. Those who are conditioned might feel the lock more than those who skipped the push-ups, however, you should still feel it.

So you are still in your 'hold', holding your breath, you have locked the stomach, now you have performed the circular movement with your shoulders (relaxed movement, requires no force, only motion from the joints) until you feel the lock – back at the original starting point. Once you have felt the lock, maintain the 'hold' for three seconds, and then lock the solar plexus, i.e., tense it as you would in one release. 'Hold' it for three seconds, then exhale, maintaining the locks until the lungs are empty. Slow-release.

It is not as complicated as it sounds. If you are finding difficulty, seek the *simplicity* and subtlety of the description and movement in Figure Seven.

Look at Figure Seven and let's review the 'one-lock' foundation technique:

1. Sit as you would in 'nafas dalam'. Focus your eyes in one direction on the flame
2. Body relaxed, back straight
3. Keep your stomach in the 'in' position
4. Inhale slowly as you would in one release, on 'hold', tense your lower stomach muscles
5. After three seconds, rotate your shoulders 360 degrees in a circular motion from a relaxed position, very gently, no force required, just move them slightly away from you, and then upwards, downwards behind you, as much as they can go, in a circular motion until they reach the original starting point, a little further, and you feel the chest muscle 'lock' into place – the shoulders here are just mechanism to lock the chest. Do this slowly first, then as you get the hang of it, do it fairly rapidly.
6. Hold it for three seconds, then lock (tense) the solar plexus
7. Hold it for three seconds, and exhale, very slowly maintaining all locks throughout

8. Repeat, up to ten times. Try holding the locks for longer, each time

FIGURE 7

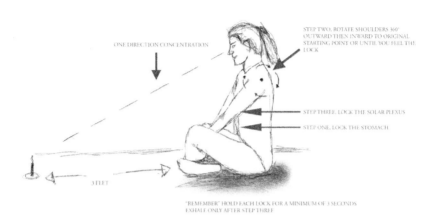

ONE DIRECTION CONCENTRATION

STEP TWO, ROTATE SHOULDERS 360° OUTWARD THEN INWARD TO ORIGINAL STARTING POINT OR UNTIL YOU FEEL THE LOCK

STEP THREE, LOCK THE SOLAR PLEXUS

STEP ONE, LOCK THE STOMACH

3 FEET

"REMEMBER" HOLD EACH LOCK FOR A MINIMUM OF 3 SECONDS
EXHALE ONLY AFTER STEP THREE

So, we have discussed the science behind central power, the advanced breathing techniques, the physical exercises and the beginnings of the 'one-lock' system.

Once you have mastered the first three locks (stomach, chest, solar plexus), keep doing it over and over, you should feel the benefits and it should make you want to repeat it, if you don't feel it, re-read, study it and re-apply. Eventually it will come to you. You can train anywhere, at home, work, you can apply the lock technique. Train the one-lock technique every day, if you are ill, elderly, disabled, apply these methods instantly, and keep repeating them, ten, twenty and more repetitions a day.

To know if you are doing it correctly, you should feel an intense focus during the exercise with your eyes focused on the flame (or dot). It is better to have less disturbance around the focal point, in order to maximize the connection to your CNS. You should feel your stomach muscles lock into place, with your chest, your solar plexus, as you keep repeating the exercises, the effects should be felt more and more. You can then apply the exercises anywhere at any time.

Keep trying, keep applying, take what you can from each of the next three chapters to turn your life around, if you are sick, elderly, or an athlete. If you are a coach, apply it to your students, on top of your own training. Then focus on this chapter in great detail, study it, practice it. The methods described in this chapter are adaptable to various sports and disciplines, but being *authentic* to your training will yield you better results. Since writing this book, I have gone back to the foundation techniques to make sure that I am describing them correctly, the results were incredible, far more Central Power was generated.

Central Power requires calm concentration, no adrenaline or emotions, to achieve the best results. What you have learnt is the first step. If you would like to learn more, contact me directly.

'I am not teaching you anything, I just help you to explore yourself.'
-*Bruce Lee*

PHYSICAL FORTITUDE

'A teacher is never a giver of truth - he is a guide, a pointer to the truth that each student must find for himself. A good teacher is merely a catalyst.'
-Bruce Lee

The benefits of physical activity *far outweigh* the 'benefits' of physical inactivity.
Research data available from the U.S National Library of Medicine states clearly that 'Physical inactivity is a modifiable risk factor for cardiovascular disease and a widening variety of other chronic diseases, including diabetes mellitus, cancer (colon and breast), obesity, hypertension, bone and joint diseases (osteoporosis and osteoarthritis), and depression'.

Both men and women who reported increased levels of physical activity and fitness were found to have reductions in relative risk (by about 20%–35%). Recent investigations have revealed even greater reductions in the risk of death from any cause and from cardiovascular disease. For instance, being fit or active was associated with a greater than 50% reduction in risk.

The benefits of physical activity and fitness extend to patients with established cardiovascular disease. This is important because, for a long time, rest and physical inactivity had been recommended for patients with heart disease. Both aerobic and resistance types of exercise have been shown to be associated with a decreased risk of type 2 diabetes. In a large prospective study, each increase of 500 kcal (2100 kJ) in energy expenditure per week was associated with a decreased incidence of type 2 diabetes of 6%.

Similarly, research is suggesting the same for Osteoporosis, Cancer and other life-threatening, debilitating, diseases and conditions.

How much exercise is enough? Research has revealed that regular physical activity (expending > 2000 kcal (calories) per week) is associated with an average increase in life expectancy of one to two years by the age of eighty. Subsequent studies have shown that an average energy expenditure of about 1000 kcal per week is associated with a 20%–30% reduction in all-cause mortality.

The research goes on, and on. However, this book is not a scientific journal. This book should give you enough reason to want to get up and take that walk, or wake up early and commit to that run, to go back into the gym, take up that class you always said you would.

The key point we can learn here is that number of calories (kcal) burned every week is a crucial factor. The rate at which people are being diagnosed with the aforementioned illnesses is staggering. It is like a lottery, luck of the draw, who is next to be diagnosed with Cancer, or Diabetes due to an unhealthy lifestyle, unfortunately.

To develop 'Central Power', you *must* one must understand that Physical Activity, daily, weekly, is a *must-do*. Our lives are consumed with chores, errands, work, business, family, each one sipping the energy from us bit by bit, leaving little left for exercise – thus the *mind* – is the crucial element here.

No one can force you to get up, not only that, the cost associated with paying for a personal trainer is not always affordable to us. You have to train your mind to take that half an hour everyday as a minimum, to do some kind of intense activity. It has to be hard-wired into the circuitry of your brain, into your routine, if you work, have a family, then it is possible for example to invest in a spinning bike, go to that class or use a fitness video and work out at home. There is always a solution.

Think about your health, your children, your family, you are doing this not just for yourself, but for them too. With all due respect to all those gravely ill, sometimes we don't have a choice, and I respect that, but those that do, need to make it now.

There is unquestionable evidence that regular physical activity contributes to the prevention of several chronic diseases and is associated with a reduced risk of premature death. There appears to be a relation between the volume of physical activity and health status, such that the most physically active people are at the lowest risk. However, the greatest improvements in health status are seen when people who are the *least fit* become physically active. New research by McMaster University points to another major benefit: better memory. The findings could have implications for an aging population which is grappling with the growing problem of shattering illnesses such as dementia and Alzheimer's.

Scientists have found that six weeks of intense exercise, short bouts of interval training over the course of 20 minutes - showed significant improvements in what is known as high-interference memory, which, for example, allows us to distinguish our car from another of the same make and model. The study is published in the *Journal of Cognitive Neuroscience*. The findings are important because memory performance of the study participants, who were all healthy young adults, increased over a relatively *short period of time*, say researchers. They also found that participants who experienced greater fitness gains also experienced greater increases in brain-derived neurotrophic factor (BDNF), a protein that supports the growth, function and survival of brain cells.

Such research provides fuel to the theory of Central Power, that physical activity, somehow, improves brain function, that this formidable organ we all have, has untapped potential to perform better, provide us with more abilities, to help us nurture and grow, Central Power delivery. Further research, in the British Medical Journal states that worldwide, 3.2 million deaths are being attributed to inactivity, annually. Physical activity is like medicine to older adults. The research states, 'in industrialized countries where people are living longer lives, the levels of chronic health conditions are increasing and the levels of physical activity are declining. Key factors in improving health are exercising at a moderate-to-vigorous level for *at least 5 days per week* and including both aerobic and strengthening exercises'.

This chapter will explore which physical exercises are the most beneficial to you, which has worked for me and are the right foundations for a base-regime training programme. We all lead hectic lifestyles and it is difficult to remain consistent in the twelve months of a year, however, certain exercises can and should be maintained, even through lulls in training. I refer to these as 'base-regime exercises'. Subsequently, as you train throughout the year, you can alter your regime as recommended by a personal trainer, new exercises you learn, classes etc. In terms of exercise, 'change' is good. Once you have a regime, and you have learnt the basics of Central Power, you can apply the techniques to your physical activity.

The first base-regime exercise I would advise, is a cardiovascular exercise such as running, jogging, or skipping, brisk walking, or even *just* walking. Whichever is in your ability. I would advise to complete the activity outdoors, regardless of the weather. If you must use a treadmill, or equivalent, set the gradient to 1% to match the energy consumed outdoors.

If you run outside, particularly if you go off-road, there is inevitably going to be more variety. Each step will be different from the one before, simply because you are running on an uneven and varied surface. Research suggests that this constant challenge not only strengthens the ligaments and activates a greater variety of muscles, but also improves your sense of balance. That said, the belt of a treadmill can be more forgiving than a hard pavement, which is important if you are carrying an injury.
Research from the University of Exeter concluded that exercising in natural environments, particularly green spaces, 'was associated with greater feelings of revitalization and positive engagement, decreases in tension, confusion, anger and depression, and increased energy'. Research also suggested that people who did exercise outdoors, enjoyed it more, had more satisfaction, and were more likely to do it again. Depending on the time of year and time that you train, there is a greater chance of exposure to Vitamin D.

I had the opportunity to train in Indonesia, where eighty percent of the time it was outdoors, either in the city, or in the mountainous regions, under waterfalls, and on the beach by the sea. Training for an hour in those conditions, was breath-taking and, if I may say so, life changing. The more you train your body for physical activities, the longer you can spend exerting yourself to train Central Power, which in turn will deliver more results.

Indoors, I recommend cycling or spinning, research has also suggested that the effect on heart rate as well as the calories burnt are greater indoors for cycling than they are when you do the same exercise outside.

Stretching is important here, before, during and after your session, and each depends on the need of the individual. Personally I stretch before, a very brief static stretch because experimenting has led me to realize I perform better and run more comfortably when I stretch before a run. However, my real stretching comes at the end, which I will discuss later. For some people, a five minute warm up may be required to prevent any muscle strain from stretching.

I run what many may consider to be long distances, usually, 8 or 4 miles, sometimes every day, sometimes on alternate days. I keep my times steady, and always try to improve on them run by run. My times also indicate to me where I am on my performance, i.e. pace per mile and kcals burned. It can be a good indicator of your overall wellbeing, and provides a new challenge every time you run.
The key element here – is to *move*. If you can't run, then jog, if you can't do that, then brisk walk, if you can't do that, then gentle walking is fine to start – or even cycling indoors. How long you exercise for is up to you, some people can do a full hour, some more, or less.

What you need to aim for is consistency, hard wiring the brain, that on this time, on this day, *you* will *move*. You could possibly even dance, jog on the spot, all depends on your abilities and desires – to achieve the outcome we want, which is successfully performing a vigorous exercise for at least 150 minutes a week, minimum.

When you go to a gym, a personal trainer can give you a great work out that gets your heart rate pumping, or you can attend a boxercise class etc. These are great and provide the results we want. Personally, I prefer to run outdoors, because it sets the base for me for my next exercises, stretching, core strength, compound exercises, and then Central Power.

Everything is about the conditions we are in, and we must adapt to the conditions. In doing so, we have to adapt to our environment, to continue our base-regime training. You don't need to be a member at a gym, to run outdoors. My current regime, purely out of choice and convenience, is a six mile run, followed by advanced Central Power or Ki exercises, that when performed daily, are the equivalent of working out with weights, without the associated side-effects. In doing so, I have attained a formidable condition, that is satisfying for myself right now. My thighs and my calves, are currently stronger than at any other time in my life, a key requirement for later stage health and fitness, which I will discuss later. However, I do intend to expand my regime with the latter mentioned exercises, purely for more results.

The next base-regime exercise I would advise, is *yoga*. According to the American Osteopathic Association, 'The purpose of yoga is to create strength, awareness and harmony in *both the mind and body*,' explains Natalie Nevins, a board-certified osteopathic family physician and certified Kundalini Yoga instructor in Hollywood, California.

The relaxation techniques in Yoga can lessen chronic pain, arthritis, headaches and carpel tunnel syndrome, lower blood pressure and reduce insomnia. Physical benefits include, improved flexibility, protection from injury, increased muscle strength and tone, improved respiration, energy and vitality, balanced metabolism, weight reduction, cardio and circulatory health, and improved athletic performance.

Yoga's incorporation of meditation and breathing can help improve a person's mental well-being. 'Regular yoga practice creates mental clarity and calmness; increases body awareness; relieves chronic stress patterns; relaxes the mind; centers attention; and sharpens concentration,' says Dr. Nevins. All are required and beneficial to begin developing Central Power.

I perform Yoga immediately after a run, before Central Power exercises. On days when I do not run, I would perform Yoga, combined with my stretches, after my Central Power exercises. I am not an expert in Yoga, the world of Yoga is full of wonderful teachers, I have picked up my favorite poses that are useful to me and that I feel, are the most beneficial for my base-regime training to develop Central Power.

The types of poses I would perform are (immediately after a run):
Child's pose or Bālāsana. Child's Pose helps to stretch the hips, thighs, and ankles while reducing stress and fatigue. It gently relaxes the muscles at the front of the body while softly and passively stretching the muscles of the back torso. From this position I would go into:
Table pose to perform the cow pose or Bitilasana - to the cat pose or Marjyasana, for an inhale and exhale. Note, once

you learn the foundations for Central Power, you can apply them to your Yoga Poses.

From this position, I would go into:

Bhujangasana or Cobra Pose is a back-bending yoga asana. It stretches muscles in the shoulders, chest and abdominals, decreases stiffness of the lower back, strengthens the arms and shoulders, increases flexibility, elevates mood, firms and tones the buttocks, relieves stress and fatigue, opens the chest and helps to clear the passages of the heart and lungs, improves circulation of blood and oxygen, especially throughout the spinal and pelvic regions.

From this position, I return to Child's Pose with hands outstretched in front of me. I remain in each pose for approximately thirty or so seconds.

From Child's Pose I would go into:

Ūrdhva Mukha Śvānāsana or Upward Facing Dog Pose. This pose improves posture, strengthens the spine, arms, wrists, stretches the chest and lungs, shoulders, and abdomen, firms the buttocks, stimulates abdominal organs, helps relieve mild depression, fatigue, and sciatica.

From Upward Facing Dog Pose, I go into:

Adho Mukha Śvānāsana or Downward-facing Dog Pose. This pose energizes and rejuvenates the entire body. It deeply stretches your hamstrings, shoulders, calves, arches, hands, and spine while building strength in your arms, shoulders, and legs.

From this moment onwards, I go into my normal, static stretching routine for my calves, quads etc.

These types of poses, are part of my base-regime, that strengthen my posture, balance and ability to generate Central Power for longer.

The next base-regime exercise I would like to discuss is, Core Development. A strong-core is imperative for successful Central Power delivery, the two exercises go hand in hand. As you train your core, and practice the foundation breathing exercises, you will feel your core becoming sturdier, around the solar plexus and the lower stomach muscles. Both have to be strong, to generate Central Power. So having Core development as a base-regime exercise, makes sense.

The benefits of training the core are numerous. Core training strengthens the muscles in your abdomen and lower back, reducing strain and back pain. It improves your posture, making you feel and look leaner and more confident. It improves your functional strength, making mundane jobs easier, i.e. housework, etc. It improves balance and overall sports performance by stabilizing your body.

There are numerous core workouts that you could do. Personal trainers incorporate theses into their regimes, gyms have core classes, learn your favourite ones and master them. Here I will discuss the core exercises I would normally perform, after my run, and yoga stretch, prior to performing my advanced Central Power techniques. I can't emphasize to you enough, the benefits of Central Power once you have strengthened your core, at the end of a workout, you should feel the results as you train.
Again, as I mentioned earlier, once you learn the foundation breathing techniques for Central Power, you can incorporate them into your core workout.

My core workout would include use of the medicine ball & swiss ball, two pieces of equipment that provide as much benefit, if not more, than weights.

Gyms have great personal trainers, that provide solutions based on you as a person, often I would work out in the gym and the personal trainer without knowing my history would raise an eyebrow at seeing me workout, I am like a hurricane. I do not believe in long rests during a workout, or stopping to have a conversation, but that's my personal choice. In the workout I have described so far, the most I would rest is ten to fifteen seconds, or take a breather in my Yoga poses, or slow down my run, adaptability and versatility are your best friends, listen to your body, train the best way that suits *your* physiology.

Rest is for bedtime, or when you finally put your feet up with your family, you will appreciate that time more when you work out. One of my closest friends, is a great ladies man, every woman he has ever met has been from the gym, the gym I guess can be a great place for that, but if you are focused on your workout, you will make *no* friends. The Monk Life, is the *life of a fighter*, the life of a fighter, is a lonely place. We are taking the best elements here to help *you*, achieve your health goals.

My sets would consist of six sets, with maximum repetitions, until I felt the pain and couldn't continue. In between each set I would rest for a maximum of thirty seconds, usually around fifteen, the pain would be intense after each set, but it should dissipate quickly, if it doesn't, stop training and speak to a specialist to check your technique.
Work your way up, if you are a beginner start slow, focus on hard wiring your brain, if you are committing to the routine, that *is* enough, time will improve your technique, rushing in, will cause injury and set you back. In Indonesia, my teacher used to say, '*slow, but sure*'. I got the gist of what he meant, and it should apply to you too.
My core workout included:

The Plank and Side-Plank, to strengthen the abdominals. Usually for around 30-60 seconds, each set.

Medicine Ball Squat (painful). Usually with the heaviest medicine ball I could find, holding it out in front of me, feet hip width apart, lower yourself until you are almost seated, and then back up again.

One handed push-ups on Swiss Ball. With my legs spread apart, one hand behind my back, and one on the center of the ball, I would try to get as many push-ups as I can out, and then switch to the other hand. This will strengthen your core like no other (in my personal experience), if you can manage this, well done, you can probably have this as your lone core exercise, it is *that* rewarding.

Knee Raisers on Swiss Ball. With the palms of my hands pressed firmly on the fitness ball (not elbows), in a semi-push-up position, I would raise one knee at a time, until the pain became unbearable.

Hanging & Weighted Knee-raisers. From the chin-up bar, using a Swiss ball, or medicine ball between the legs, usually you need someone to help you with this one.

Swiss Ball Sit-ups.

Various Kettle-bell exercises.

Weighted sit-ups (not for beginners). My personal favorite. On the adjustable abdominal board, which is where your feet are locked and you lay in a decline position – used by bodybuilders for decline dumbbell press, I would lay in a sit-up position with either a twenty or twenty-five kilogram weight on my abdominals, and do 6 sets until the pain became unbearable.

The above is what works for me, there are a wealth of core exercises that you can utilize, pick the best of what works for you. If you are a beginner, take a core class at your gym, however the above exercises, if you can master them, are in my experience what help strengthen the core and make Central Power delivery that much easier.

The next, and last base-regime exercises I would like to discuss are Compound Exercises. These exercises offer numerous benefits that help you in the real world, and ultimately improve your Central Power. They burn more calories in less time, using more muscles, improve coordination, reaction time and balance, decrease the risk of injury in sports, increase your heart rate during the work out providing you with cardiovascular benefits, they allow you to lift heavier loads and build more strength.

You can apply the foundation breathing techniques to build Central Power to these exercises, however, personally I do not. The reason being is that, modern training has advanced and has its benefits, so following the recommendations for breathing, particularly in these exercises is paramount. In addition, we are saving Central Power for the last workout, where you will see as you practice, every muscle you have worked out from these methods as described, is being worked out internally with the Central Power techniques. I call them, the *internal*-muscles.

There are numerous Compound Exercises that you can do. The ones that I would apply to my workout are:

The Deadlift.

The Bench Press.

The Squat.

Pull-ups – wide armed.

The Dip.

The Clean & Press.

I would perform them at my heaviest weight, and try to get at least two repetitions out, if not more, with a slightly longer rest in between, around sixty seconds. These will help boost growth hormone and testosterone in your body, which has numerous health benefits, there is no need for performance enhancing drugs, if you eat, train, and live right. If I had to pick one, because in my workout, you would be tired by the time you reach this point, with perhaps just enough energy for one – I would pick the deadlift by far.

So, we have discussed the importance of physical activity on your health, the base-regime exercises in this chapter that help build the foundations to develop Central Power in the first chapter. In review, these are – running, yoga, core development, compound exercises, in one workout before applying Central Power techniques to your body. These base-regime exercises are ones you should maintain throughout the year, if you have periods where you don't go to the gym, there is something you can always do, as your foundation.

The benefits of this are numerous, and I am trying to get the reader to a point where he or she can find his Central Power easily – if you were to get a boxer and teach them the techniques, he or she would see results quickly, because his mind and body are already in the right condition to achieve it. That is not to say if you do not apply it, you won't see it. We can't expect the elderly, frail, sick to work out like this, nor can we expect someone to become an athlete overnight. I have merely applied my workout, for the reader to take what he or she can, within their *own* boundaries to help them, achieve Central Power.

Physical activity is not the only requirement for Central Power, it is just one foundation, the ones who can concentrate the longest, have the best chance. When I trained in Indonesia, I came across many old masters of Ki, or Central Power, none had protruding muscles or bodies of Greek Gods, they were mere men or women, in sight, that

held an inner strength, that could be seen from their eyes –
the most important tool – to help you develop Central
Power. This chapter, is your *catalyst*, to getting you to be
physically active, if you are not already, in the best way
possible to develop your 'Inner Fortitude'.

'If you spend too much time thinking about a thing, you will
never get it done. Make at least one definite move daily
toward your goal'.
-Bruce Lee

MENTAL FORTITUDE

'As you think, so shall you become.'
-Bruce Lee

In order for you to begin developing Central Power, your mind has to be 'fit'. This is because of the amount of concentration required, as you will learn later.

That doesn't mean that someone who struggles with mental health, or with the inability to concentrate for long periods would be incapable of developing Central Power. Because as we will see here, there are methods available to us to help train ourselves, our brain, our minds, to do what we *want* it to do.

A study by the University of Manchester has shown that self-harm among teenage girls has risen 68% in three years. The findings showed that youngsters who self-harmed were about nine times more likely to die an unnatural death than those who did not, seventeen times more likely to die from suicide and thirty four times more likely to die from acute alcohol or drug poisoning.

My aim is not to alarm you. If you are a young adult, teenager, or parent of a young child struggling with mental health, the great thing is you are reading this book and taking the *first steps* to improvement. Mental health services are lacking in funding to cope with the demand, twelve mental health bodies in the U.K. wrote an open letter to the Government urging ministers that 'they cannot go-on' with so many patients 'locked-out' of vital services.

Do you want to be one of those patients who are 'locked out'? Some of us do not have a choice, some mental illnesses are genetic, or so severe, professional intervention is needed. Others, if your mental health is at the cusp of depression, panic attacks, anxiety, or something else, lingering, you would find yourself with perhaps, a lot of the population. The old adage is true, 'be careful how you treat someone, we often do not know what battle they are fighting'. The hardest fights, are inside us, kept secret from those around us, and those closest to us.

I have had first-hand experience with Schizophrenia, Huntington's disease, Alzheimer's and Dementia. My heart goes out to all the sufferers.

This book, is not meant to be a miracle, but if your mental health verses mental illness is a line, and what you learn in here pushes you closer to mental health, even if it's just 5%, then it is a success. If you keep applying, the 5% could become 7%, and so on. Additionally, applying the *whole* programme of the book to your life, The Monk Life, will undoubtedly bring further improvements.

In order for you to achieve Central Power, you must be able to focus. The inability to focus, is a weakness to work on. People who suffer from mental illness, either mild or severe, and therefore perhaps find it hard to focus, must practice through therapy and self-control. Additionally, the methods in here will help you overcome your mental illness, perhaps through the help of a counsellor or therapist, or for the more resilient, on your own.

That being said, I have seen people who suffer from anxiety and depression, who are still able to focus – in that case they can still practice the foundation breathing techniques for Central Power, which will alleviate some of the *milder* symptoms.

More people than ever before are suffering from mental and emotional distress, according to a new study. Many lack access to adequate treatment, despite legislation implemented over the last ten years designed to reduce these gaps in health coverage. The study, published in the journal of Psychiatric Services, used data from census interviews to estimate that 3.4% of the U.S. population, or more than eight million Americans, suffer from 'serious psychological distress' or SPD, a term used to describe feelings of sadness, worthlessness, and restlessness that are hazardous enough to impair physical wellbeing.

The aim in this chapter is to provide you with solutions to train your mind, many of which worked for me. In addition, the chapter is not a sole solution - physical exercise and nutrition are paramount for your mental health. Physical exercise releases the hormones in your body that help improve physiological functions such as blood sugar levels, muscle repair and growth and brain function.

Neurotransmitters known as endorphins are also released – these are natural opiates which elevate your mood helping to reduce depression and anxiety. Squats, dead-lifts and bench press are known to elevate testosterone and growth hormone levels, hormones crucial for mental health. Many depressive states men face can also be a cause of Andropause (male menopause), caused by a drop in testosterone levels. Over consumption of caffeine can lead to anxiety and panic attacks. As we get older, our physiology changes, and we find that what we could have consumed, partaken in etc., ten years ago, is no longer the same, therefore we must adapt to our physiology, and learn from our body, looking for the signs, and the symptoms.

I used to be a heavy coffee drinker, three-shots in the morning, and then perhaps a caffeine fueled workout drink in the afternoon, and I would still be able to sleep. Nowadays, I can no longer drink coffee without suffering from insomnia, I can just about have one tea. I have *adjusted*, learnt from my body and mind, and now require less consumption to exert perhaps more energy, than I did with 'false-toxins' – supplements with varied results, that perhaps do more harm than good in the long term.

However, nutrition, *is* important, and the right natural choices for you will be discussed in the next chapter. When we develop Central Power, I asked you to focus your eyes, in one direction, without moving the pupils, if you move them, you lose. Often, we are so immersed in our daily stress, life struggles and personal problems, it is hard to concentrate, or focus. It is imperative you learn how to focus these 'triggers', internally so as to not affect you externally, i.e. causing your pupils to move due to being agitated, for example, being unable to make eye contact with a person, and so on.

My aim is not to *cure* your depression, anxiety or other mental illnesses, but to be the catalyst that helps *you* take the right steps for you to deal with your mental health. There are many techniques, some work better for one person than for others. Trial and error is key. Experiment, learn, report, *conclude*.

Let's start with some of the easier ways to improve your mental health and focus, which will in turn help you develop more Central Power.

Set yourself daily and weekly goals – cut the clutter in your life into small achievable goals, write these down somehow. Take on new challenges, no matter how insignificant they may seem. Even if you are unsure of how you will perform, taking it on and completing it can do wonders for your confidence.

Get enough sleep. Around six to eight hours a night, find your optimum cycle. I find mine is six, if I go to above eight, I will under-perform in the day.

Remove toxic people from your life. This can be challenging, especially if they are family members or relationships, however you have to make *you*, number one, if they are affecting your mental health. Choose your friends wisely, if your best friend is a self-harming, depressive, procrastinating, anxious person, and you are lingering in that field too, perhaps they are not the best fit. Sign-post them to who can help them or make a decision together to overcome these problems.

Find optimistic, confident people to spend time with. This also means online/on social media, avoid people who always complain, or over-hype their lifestyles. Even if they won't engage with you, learn from positive and successful people, buy a book about a famous person who did well, who came from nowhere and now teaches their life story, and learn from that, like 'The Pursuit of Happiness'.

Count your blessings, every day. Be grateful for everything, no matter how small, even the imperfections, in those is a blessing too. I have a saying. 'Every person's weakness, is also their greatest strength, and vice versa'. A rule for you, if ever you needed to analyze something, or someone.

Make time for yourself. If you live a hectic lifestyle, always doing errands, chores, for others, don't forget *you*. Listen to some soothing sounds, YouTube is full of anti-anxiety, relaxing music, or you can listen to books, instead of reading them (Audible), or religious recitations, if you have a faith. Whatever soothes you, find it, use it.

Take timeout from your digital devices and stop multi-tasking. Smartphones, tablets etc. overstimulate our brains, take a digital detox every day. Stop sending emails at lunch, or even whilst on the phone. Something I am guilty of.
If you feel you suffer from anxiety or depression, seek help and advice for your mental health. Speak to your doctor, a counsellor, therapist, get their opinion, perhaps there is a medical reason, or perhaps there is nothing to worry about at all.

Check your heart rate on a regular basis, discover your resting heart rate. Find out what your 'triggers' are and try to find ways to alleviate them, such as what was mentioned above.

List your 'triggers' and solutions together, so that when they occur you have a solution, i.e. you are worried about your relationship, your anxiety increases, you find going for a ten minute stroll helps lower your heart rate and the feeling of anxiousness.

Stay away from drugs. If you have mental health problems, drugs will only make it worse, until you fix the problem don't start another problem, especially hard drugs like Cocaine, Heroin, Ecstasy, Ketamine and the latest trend of herbal, legal highs which are known to have taken lives. All affect our vulnerable state of mind in some way; the brain is your most valued organ and pathway to Central Power, playing with it whilst you are mentally weak will lead you down the road to further weaknesses that will be harder to alleviate.

Nourish your social life, as mentioned earlier, if you don't have people you can connect to, join community groups, force yourself to get up and join that group, like a book club or sports team.

Confiding in others and listening to similar experiences can help to relieve burden. Find peers to speak to, from your friends who are close or far and confide in them. Join online support groups or forums, consisting of people who you are struggling like you with their mental health and seeking support.

Now let's move onto the more therapeutic ways to improve your mental health. This information should serve as a catalyst for you to seek the right method for you, be it alone or through one of the wonderful therapists that work in this sector. In my opinion, *both* methods are great, especially a private therapist or counsellor if you can afford it – if not, then register with your Doctor as soon as possible to get on the waiting list, which in the U.K. is around two to three months. You should use *every* available resource to work on your *most* valuable asset, your mind, your brain, your mental health.

Mindfulness. Mindfulness is a technique which can help people manage their mental health or simply gain more enjoyment from life. It involves making a special effort to give your full attention to what is happening in the *present moment* – to what is happening in your body, your mind or your surroundings, for example – in a non-judgmental way. Mindfulness describes a way of approaching our thoughts and feelings so that we become more aware of them and react differently to them.

Mindfulness has been adapted into structured programmes – like mindfulness-based stress reduction (MBSR) in the 1970s and then mindfulness-based cognitive therapy (MBCT) – to help people manage long term health conditions and enhance their general wellbeing.

Mindfulness can help you to increase the awareness of your thoughts and feelings. Remember, it is *your* mind, *your* imagination, ultimately, *you* control everything. It can help you develop more helpful responses to difficult feelings and events, be kinder to yourself, feel calmer and able to manage stress better. It can help you manage a physical health problem such as chronic pain.

It is not *that* easy to do and requires *Mind Power*. As Bruce Lee said, 'as you think, so shall you become'. Practice makes perfect. You will have to find what works for you. Sometimes a bit of everything works, sometimes just one technique is a game changer. What is important is the effort and time you put in, consistency and determination. The results are important but if you do not yield the positive results straight away, try a different method.

In mindfulness you try to become more aware of your thoughts, emotions and physical feelings. This can help you notice when you get caught up in negative thoughts, so that you can manage them and become aware of the effect that thoughts or events have on your body, so that you can look after yourself, thus feel able to make a choice about how you respond to your thoughts and feelings. You can observe these thoughts coming and going and do not have to define who you are or your experience of the world. Ultimately, your thoughts, are *your* choice – remember, they are 'just thoughts', they can leave your mind just as easily as they entered.

If you are upset over the past, worrying about the future, you have to learn to *'let go'* and live in the present. Make the *choice*. Mindfulness trains you to create space between the negative feelings and you, focusing your mind on an alternative sensation. For this it is also useful, to start practicing Central Power.

For this type of mindfulness you can apply the foundation breathing techniques for Central Power, whilst focusing your pupils in one direction, focus on other sensations in or around you, away from the negativity. For example, the sound and length of your breathing, a noise around you, perhaps of flowing water.

This brings me to negative feelings and imagination. We all suffer from negative thoughts and emotions, it's how we repel them that makes us different. Your mind, is *your* mind, *you* control *your* imagination. If an overwhelming thought persistently interrupts you, turn the thought into something physical in your mind, make yourself something stronger than that thought, face it and destroy it. It may not work for everyone, but it may works for some of us, especially children. The saying goes, 'repel evil, with good'. The same should be applied to thoughts, repel negative thoughts, with positive thoughts. Make it your remedy, your medication, every time the thought appears in your mind. For example, a negative thought appears, you turn into a fighter, you are in the other corner and 'you knock it out of the ring'. You could turn it into a baseball and hit a home run out of the stadium. You may have to repeat the process, but that will only encourage your brain to hard wire the repelling process into the circuitry.

Cognitive Behavioral Therapy (CBT) is another, recommended method to improve your mental health. CBT is a type of talking therapy that focuses on how your thoughts, beliefs and attitudes affect your feelings and behavior, and teaches you coping skills for dealing with different problems.

It examines the things you think (cognitive therapy) and the things you do (behavior therapy), examining, the 'self-critic' within us. 'Self-talk', how we talk to ourselves, can be extremely damaging. The aim should be for you to alter your inner-voice, to make it optimistic, fulfilling, kinder and powerful, repelling your self-critic, and ordering your brain to do what you want it to do, including thoughts, feelings and emotions, *choosing* the right *feeling*.

CBT is based around the idea that how we think about situations can affect the way we think and behave. For example, if you interpret a situation negatively, then you might experience negative emotions as a result, and those bad feelings might lead you to behave in a certain way. It assumes, and I think rightfully so in many cases, that negative thinking arose from childhood, i.e. from parents or teachers who didn't praise you enough, leading you to tell yourself, 'I'm useless', or 'I'm not good enough'. Overtime these feelings become automatic and encroach into your adulthood, work, relationships, etc.

In CBT, you work with a therapist to identify and challenge any negative thinking patterns and behavior which may be causing you difficulty. In turn, this can change the way you feel about situations and enable you to change your behavior in future.

You and your therapist may look at life in the present, as well in the past, and think about how your past experiences impact how you see the world.

CBT is a relatively flexible therapy that can adapt to meet your needs. The National Institute for Health and Care Excellence (NICE), particularly recommends CBT for depression and anxiety, as well as drug related issues, relationships, insomnia, post-traumatic stress disorder, obsessive compulsive disorder, phobias, psychosis, schizophrenia and general, chronic health problems. It is a short-term solution, usually around twelve one hour sessions, once a week, you will be tasked with a lot of writing, usually one on one, or in a group. Finding a therapist, one that you connect with, can do wonders for your mental health.

Hypnotherapy. Hypnotherapy is a form of complementary therapy that utilizes the power of *positive suggestion* to bring about subconscious change to our thoughts, feelings and behavior.

The process itself aims to alter our state of consciousness in a way that relaxes the conscious part of the mind while simultaneously stimulating and focusing the subconscious part. This heightened state of awareness - reached using skilled relaxation techniques - allows the therapist to then make appropriate suggestions.

While more concrete evidence is needed to support the use of hypnosis in additional areas as an alternative to conventional medicine, many have found the process has been incredibly effective either when used in tandem with traditional treatment or when used independently after other avenues have been exhausted.

Visit a Hypnotherapists' website and have a read of the testimonials, of all the people who have overcome certain conditions, be it phobias or anxiety. Hypnotherapy is widely gaining steam in the medical world as a recognized therapy, having been recently recommended by NICE as a treatment for Irritable Bowel Syndrome.

A typical therapist will not usually see you for more than three or four sessions, as they describe it as a 'fast-fix', unless you wanted more. A session will involve opening up about your personal life and medical issues, your goals and problems, and what kind of solution orientated hypnotherapy you require.

It has been known to be effective in the treatment of addictions, anger management, anxiety, depression, eating disorders, low confidence, obsessions and compulsions, pain disorders, post-traumatic stress disorder, relationships, insomnia, stress, sports, public speaking, stuttering, weight loss and so on.

There are different types of Hypnotherapy, such as Neuro-linguistic Hypnotherapy (NLP). NLP is regarded as a tool-kit for the mind, used to improve many areas of a person's life. It focuses on the future, exploring it's possibilities and solutions, rather than looking into past experiences. NLP encourages individuals to challenge themselves and take chances.

Suggestive hypnotherapy, is a 'suggestion' a hypnotherapist will place into your subconscious to positively influence your thoughts and behaviors, i.e. for stopping smoking, or for reducing anxiety, to *improve self-talk.* If your self-critic is extreme and damaging, I would highly recommend hypnotherapy to reverse this, and help you to think and be more optimistic. You will be surprised at how the 'positive-you' can benefit yourself and those around you.

Some people are more susceptible to suggestion than others, factors that contribute to success are your willingness, your dedication to the therapy and your trust and bond with the therapist.

It can clear the clutter in your mind and leave you thinking 'efficiently' with your brain; all the elements required to deliver Central Power.

Solution-focused hypnotherapy looks at your present situation, and your future. It makes you set concrete, specific and realistic goals for the future. Once you have done this, your therapist will use questioning techniques to identity your preferred future, making solutions more obvious, giving you actionable steps to take in order to reach your goal. A core belief of this type of hypnotherapy is that *you,* have the strength and resources to solve your own problems, the role of the therapist is merely to prompt and guide you.

There are so many solution and suggestive based hypnotherapies, available for download or online, or from a great, local therapist. Perhaps you could experiment with one or two downloads, listen to the recording, and then make your decision.

Clearing clutter in your mind, believing in yourself, your actions, repelling negative thoughts, creating a positive self-talk inside you, all enhance the ability to *focus*.

Focus, is the key to developing Central Power. The Monk Life, that I try to live daily, has so far described to you ways to improve your physical health dramatically, ways to improve your mental health, and work towards a complete solution to mind, body & soul.

Having a clear mind, can enhance every other area of your life, it will improve your focus in training, in your day to day tasks, and in family life. People will slowly start to notice the change. But these changes will only take place when *you*, make the right choices, applying the effort required to achieve them. Nothing happens, when you procrastinate, 'things' do not fall on to your lap and give you a 'quick-fix' or 'magic-solution'.

I can understand, when depression hits, anxiety hits, it's almost like the will to live leaves your body, the will *to do*, to *achieve* goes, and a powerful, athletic person becomes a weakling. Physical strength is not a sign of having excellent mental health.

This is when you have to talk to yourself, you have to create a stronger you, inside you, to defeat the self-critic. Training the mind to do what you want it to do, to make the right choices. Spending a hundred pounds on the weekend, on alcohol, junk food, taxis and that new date for a temporary fix, or paying for two counselling, therapy sessions that will send you into a more productive week and possibly change your life.

If you are addicted to drugs, the choice could be between spending that fifty pounds on a gram of cocaine, or on your first hypnotherapy session to get you off the addiction. Work out how much money you could save by quitting drugs, cigarettes, alcohol and spend it in *your* cause, the cause of your mental and physical health.

This cannot be said enough, set goals every day. Put aside a money-box, and every day put in your small change, every time you suffer from anxiety, depression, a phobia, or something else, put money in the tin. Why? Because until you do something about it, it will continue to cost you, cost your learning, cost your development, cost your progress, cost your health, your friends, family, everyone you care for. The money in the tin will build up and pay for your first private therapy session.

There is a saying, 'do not rest on your laurels', the saying rings true. If you leave these lingering problems, they build up slowly, become worse and diminish your ability to achieve in the future. In this case they will diminish your chances of developing Central Power. Be grateful, if they are lingering problems and strike now while you can. If they are severe episodes, seek professional help immediately, get that support network around you, if it's not available, perhaps create it, online or in a community group.
They say, what you put in to the world, you will get back, so go out there and help someone, *serve* them, feed the homeless or counsel someone suffering from depression and anxiety, volunteer in a home for the elderly, etc. Take them this book and teach them the foundation breathing techniques. The little things you do for others, will encourage your mental health to improve by helping you to feel better about yourself. Find a purpose that will help you

live a meaningful life, be it volunteering, or just helping your elderly neighbour once a week.

Expect things to work, if you work out, or take a supplement, or go to therapy, expect the best. Research suggests that the 'placebo' affect influences the effect of the treatment we undergo.

Being positive in situations, regardless of the outcome, is a strong, positive trait to possess. There is a blessing in everything, sometimes we just don't see it. Remaining steadfast and strong, gives you power over everything, nothing or no one can hurt you. Why? Because you will remain disciplined, with inner-strength and *inner fortitude*. Be grateful and destroy your self-critic. Tell yourself every day, 'I choose to be strong', or 'I choose to be content', 'I choose to be secure'. Positive *orders* to yourself can have a rewarding effect on how your mind regulates emotions, in the end no matter what happens, *you* are in control.
If you feel anxious, say 'I choose to let go of all anxiety', if you feel angry, 'I choose to forgive'. You can say, 'I choose to smile', 'I choose to be happy', so on and so forth. Close your eyes, talk to yourself, be your own strength in your mind. Re-programme the brain, every day, re-wire your circuitry to be kinder to yourself, to others, to your *family*. Fight the negative thoughts, *imagine* the fight in your mind, and win the battle.

Choose to be optimistic, say it to yourself every day, 'I choose to be optimistic', it works wonders for you and being optimistic has shown to boost your immune system. Writing a gratitude journal before you sleep encourages a good night's sleep. Write about the small things that made you happy and content today, make them powerful.

Remember the old saying, it takes only a little good, to destroy something a lot more evil.

Listen to brainwave sounds. Studies have shown that there is enough effectiveness to warrant further research. Developing Central Power is a form of meditation. Numerous studies have shown that meditation slows the rate of cellular aging, helps you to remain youthful, helps ward-off age related diseases, boosts your immune system and improves your emotional wellbeing. Start meditating now, before you learn the foundation breathing techniques, as preparation for something even *more* powerful. Remember, we are connecting the mind and the body to develop Central Power, and in order to do so we must prepare it in the best condition possible for us. We are only humans and not perfect, the important thing is to believe in yourself, believe in your abilities, and push through the days when you will fail. Failure is not the end, failure is just the beginning. When you battle to concentrate, remember that you are *trying*, when you stop, take a break for however long you want, an hour, a day, and then come back and try again. If you are consistent, you *will* progress.

'I fear not the man who has practiced ten thousand kicks. I fear the man who practiced one kick, ten thousand times'.
-Bruce Lee

NUTRITIONAL FORTITUDE

'In order to taste from my cup of water, you must first *empty* your cup'.
-*Bruce Lee*

'You must first *empty* your cup'. Read the sentence, listen to the words inside as you read them. You have to change your nutritional habits in order to achieve the perfect balance of mental, physical, internal health.

Some of us may have to scrap our diet completely and start again fresh. This may require some mental strength, if so, read the last chapter and perhaps seek help.

'*Balance*' is key here. In the developing world, over eight hundred million people suffer from chronic undernourishment, whereas both developed and emerging economies are facing rising levels of obesity and diet related disease (heart disease, type 2 diabetes, cancer, high blood pressure, osteoarthritis). Of course, these are due to changes in the pattern of consumption, as well as more sedentary lifestyles. This chapter will discuss the importance of nutritional fortitude and how to improve your nutritional intake.

Our nutrition represents the understanding of the nature and interaction of two systems: the external and internal. The external represents our food system and concerns the ability to source food from the wider environment, a complete diet providing adequate energy and nutrients. The internal, represents the body's biochemical, physiological and metabolic processes which create the optimum internal environment for cells, tissues and organs to maintain their structure and function, to ensure ongoing health. Health is protected and enabled when the two systems operate in *balance* and *harmony.*

Our nutritional requirements will vary according to age, sex, body type, genotype, level of activity, physiological status (i.e. pregnant), and the presence or absence of disease. Research indicates that optimum nutrition, from preconception through to adulthood and to later years of life plays a key role in lifelong health and healthy ageing. Our chances of developing a diet related disease can be greatly reduced or increased by the nutritional choices we make. Furthermore, changes do not happen overnight, they are the result of consistent behavioral changes, from three to six months to two years, before you can notice the difference. The concept of energy intake versus energy output, is insufficient. We have to look at quality *and* quantity. Quality is the carbohydrates, essential fatty acids, amino acids, minerals, vitamins, trace elements, water, oxygen. Quantity is the energy from macronutrients, carbohydrates, protein and fat to ensure optimal healthy growth and function. Our physical activity sets the demand for intake, therefore The Monk Life sets the criteria for physical activity *first.* Carbohydrates, fat and protein are macronutrients, that we need to eat in relatively large amounts in the diet as they provide our body with energy and the building blocks for growth and maintenance.

Vitamins and minerals are micronutrients, which are essential nutrients our body needs in *small* amounts in order to work properly. Small, yet consistent changes are the goals for us here.

Most of us are able to get the nutrients we need by following the dietary guidelines set here, but in some cases we need to supplement, for example, during pregnancy, or if suffering from Vitamin D deficiency and so on.

The basics of carbohydrates (energy), fibre (digestive health, reduces heart disease), protein (energy and amino acids, some that we can't make ourselves) and fat (essential fatty acids, that we can't make ourselves, need in small amounts and helpful for the absorption of fat-soluble vitamins) are generally well known and in our day to day diet. This chapter will discuss what we should *remove*, what we should *add*.

In terms of diet, there is no one-size fits all method, what works for you may not work for someone else. It is therefore imperative to create your own diet plan, using the knowledge you learn here, or from a nutritionist or dietician. Again trial and error is crucial to your advancement, knowing your own body, your own physiology.
One study, published in JAMA in 2007, comparing the Atkins (very low carbohydrate) diet to others has generally been inconclusive but shows favorable results for women. Some effectiveness has been shown in low fat, high protein type diets (published in The New England Journal of Medicine in 2009) which is the type I choose to follow, when necessary. Interestingly, the study also showed that those who attended counselling sessions, lost more weight and regained less, showing that behavioral, psychological and social factors are *equally* as important.

Nowadays, I eat healthy throughout the week, then let go on other days like the weekend. We are only human, 'what you put in everyday, is what you will get out'. If I put in junk daily, such as drinking fizzy drinks, eating fried food, burgers, fries etc., inevitably I will under-perform in my training, my body fat will increase, there will perhaps be some mental changes too, to my mood and wellbeing. Putting in the right food, gives you the right output in your training, better results, visibly and mentally. Meaning that you will see it, and feel it. The older you are, the less your mind and body can take *'negative food'* – the food that ultimately hurts you.

Being in shape, having tight muscles around the mid-section, i.e. lower stomach and solar plexus is essential for Central Power. Training Central Power will not burn fat unless you live in a tropical climate, nor will it provide you with adequate nutrition, The Monk Life is a total solution to creating the optimal conditions for Central Power delivery. Having excessive fat around the midsection and other parts of the body is not only detrimental to your health, but can hinder your progress. Having said that, excessive weight around the midsection will not stop you from developing Central Power. Central Power will improve your posture, pushing the belly in making you appear slimmer.
Central Power delivery requires cognitive strength, a new study by the University of Illinois, found that monounsaturated fatty acids (MUFAs), a class of nutrients found in olive oils, nuts and avocados, are linked to general intelligence. The study was published in the journal Neurolmage. The researchers found that general intelligence was associated with the brain's dorsal attention network, which plays a central role in attention-demanding tasks and everyday problem solving.

In turn, they found that those with higher levels of MUFAs in their blood had greater small-world propensity (the measure used to describe how well the neural network is connected and how efficient the dorsal attention network is) in their dorsal attention network. Taken together with an observed correlation between higher levels of MUFAs and greater general intelligence, these findings suggest MUFAs affect cognition noticeably.

Additionally, new research suggest type 2 diabetes isn't necessarily for life. A new clinical trial provides the clearest evidence yet that the condition can be reversed. A clinical trial involving 300 people in the U.K found an intensive weight management program put type 2 diabetes into remission for 86% of patients who lost fifteen kilograms or more. The participants had to restrict themselves to a low calorie formula diet consisting of things like health shakes and soups, limiting them to consuming 825-853 calories per day for a period of three to five months. After this, food was reintroduced to the diet slowly over two to eight weeks, and participants were given support to maintain their weight loss, including cognitive behavioural therapy and help with how to increase their level of physical activity. For most of the people willing to make the sacrifices, the result was worth it, almost 90% of those who lost fifteen kilograms, reversed their type 2 diabetes, and 57% of those dropping ten to fifteen kilograms also achieved remission.

More and more research is being done that shows promising results in how nutrition affects us in more than just our stomach. The time for change is *now*. No more late night pizza, unless it's your birthday, no more fizzy drinks, no more donner meat, no more food from questionable sources. Remember, everything in The Monk Life, does not just benefit you but also those around you, your family, your loved ones.

What if your lifestyle led to heart disease, you had to leave work, your family had to support you, everyone takes a hit, not just you. What if you could do something now to reduce the probability of that ever happening? We don't work on hindsight, we live in the now, there is no time machine to go back and tell you how to live, if you are reading this, make the change *now*.

Let's start by talking about what you should remove from your diet.

Sugary drinks. The most fatty aspect of the modern diet. This drives insulin resistance, and is linked to type 2 diabetes, heart disease and fatty liver disease.

Pizza. High in calories, highly refined wheat flour, and processed meat. If you must, make a homemade pizza with a thin base and wholesome ingredients. Apologies to the pizza shops.

White bread. Refined wheat is low in nutrients and leads to spikes in blood sugar.

Most fruit juices. Depending on the ingredients they could be just fruit flavored sugar-water. Opt for the healthy ones containing no added sugars and sweeteners, a hundred percent pure pomegranate or blueberry juice.

Industrial vegetable oils. Strong concern over these, as they have been linked to cancer. Opt for coconut oil or extra virgin olive oil.

Margarine. Too many artificial ingredients and trans-fat.

Pastries, cookies and cakes. High in calories, refined sugar, saturated fats and wheat. One of the worst things you can do to your body, no more cinnamon bun with that latte in the morning, note to myself there.

French fries and potato chips. Opt for boiled potatoes at restaurants or for meals at home instead of fried or other raw food alternatives such as carrot sticks etc.

Agave nectar and other high fructose alternatives. Opt for Stevia or natural honey, dates as an alternative but be wary of amounts consumed if you are diabetic.

Low-fat yoghurt. Usually contains a load of sugar, opt for full-fat that contains probiotics and reduce the intake.

Ice cream. For obvious reasons. Opt for dairy free, naturally sweetened ice cream now and then. However if you train like a hurricane, treat yourself, I would.

Candy bars. Processed and saturated fats, refined wheat and high in sugar, opt for dark chocolate with greater than 50% cocoa instead.

Processed meat. Linked to colon cancer, type 2 diabetes and heart disease.

Soy & soy protein. If you are male, these reduce your testosterone levels.

Most fast food meals. Made in the cheapest possible way with no health benefits taken into consideration. Far too much salt.

Anything high in sugar, any processed food, refined grains, vegetable oils and artificial trans-fat.

Now, removing the above from your diet may seem challenging; if you are addicted, use the mental strengthening techniques described in the last chapter to aid you. If you are obese and can't control your intake, you have to learn to fight the craves. Find stories of people who have turned their lives around, there are many out there, you will become one too.

Now let's look at what to add to your diet. Adding food to your diet can be done in several ways, as a snack, which you nibble in between meals, mix it with your main meal in your cooking, in a smoothie, whatever you choose, just get it down you. Remember the rule, small, consistent changes, will bring the best results *over time*.

People take a host of supplements on a day to day basis, hoping for some benefit, in some cases there is, in others, the pill just turns to waste. The supplement industry is worth billions, everyone wants a quick-fix, a magic pill. Sorry, but there is no Viagra for nutrition, yet.

Try food, first. The right combination of food can provide the right nutrients at the right time, for your mental and physical health. Unless you're advised against it by a physician, try investing in superfoods, fruit and nuts for a while.

Before we start, a note about antioxidants. Antioxidants come up frequently in discussions about good health and preventing diseases. These powerful substances, which mostly come from the fresh fruits and vegetables we eat, prohibit (and in some cases even prevent), the oxidation of other molecules in the body. The benefits of antioxidants are very important to good health, because if free radicals are left unchallenged, they can cause a wide range of illnesses and chronic diseases.

The human body naturally produces free radicals and the antioxidants to counteract their damaging effects. However, in most cases, free radicals far outnumber the naturally occurring antioxidants. In order to maintain the balance, a *continual supply* of external sources of antioxidants is necessary in order to obtain the maximum benefits of antioxidants. Antioxidants benefit the body by neutralizing and *removing* free radicals from the bloodstream.

Brazil nut. Lots of MOFAs, raises good cholesterol, lowers bad, contains selenium, which increases antioxidants in the body, fights heart disease and cancer.

Spinach. Ever watch Popeye? It wasn't a joke. Strengthens bones, boosts brain power with omega 3 fatty acids, fights cancer and so on.

Broccoli. Flushes cancer causing chemicals from the body, reduces tumour growth, increases cognitive function.

Walnuts. Lots of Omega 3's, which boost brain function. High in antioxidants, iron, manganese, zinc.

Garlic. Raw, one clove, crunch it, down it with water, helps prevent cancer and more.

Black pepper. Stimulate fat cell break down, contains antioxidants.

Lentils. Low calorie, high in protein, fiber, lower cholesterol, stabilize blood sugar and prevent heart disease.

Fish oil. Omega 3 fatty acids, increased cardiovascular health.

Ginger. Personal favorite. Fights off a cold, speeds up digestion, anti-cancer agent, cognitive enhancer, menstrual symptom reliever.

Grapefruit. High in vitamin C, boosts immune system, reduces heart related illnesses, including stroke and heart attack, detoxification of the liver, lowers cholesterol, reduces the chances of breast cancer. However grapefruit cannot be eaten if you are on statins and some other medications, read your patient information leaflet provided with the drugs to check.

Oats. High in fiber, reduces your chances of high blood pressure, high in antioxidants, prevent arteries from hardening, reduces the chances of breast cancer, stabilizes blood sugar levels.

Wild salmon. High in Omega 3's, improves mood, cognition, decreases risk of stroke, heart attack and high blood pressure.

Hemp seed. Contains all nine essential amino acids, and omega 6's and 3's.

Blueberries. Boosts brain power, may reduce symptoms associated with dementia, regulates blood sugar, high in antioxidants, improves learning and motor skills.

Goji berries. Another personal favorite. Contain eighteen amino acids, high in protein, hunger reducing, boosts the immune and nervous system, high in antioxidants, increase brain and muscle functionality.

Pomegranates. High in antioxidants, high in fiber, improves blood flow, slows growth of prostate cancer, reduce bad cholesterol.

Green Tea. My daily intake is at least two-three cups. High in nutrients and antioxidants, boosts the immune system, cognitive health, brain function, aids fat burning, reduces risk of cancer, twenty percent reduction in heart disease for individuals who consume four cups a day, reduces risk of Parkinson's or Alzheimer's.

Honey. Another favorite. Treatment of indigestion or acid reflux, antibacterial, boosts immune system, relief from allergies, reduces white blood cell count.

Oranges. High in vitamin C, high in fiber, helps prevent cancer, increases heart health, fights infections and regulates blood sugar.

Sweet potato. A regular meal for me. High in antioxidants, high in vitamin C and A, which helps the body repair skin and other tissues, regulates blood sugar, antifungal, boosts brain and nerve functions.

Turmeric. High in antioxidants, anti-viral, anti-inflammatory, reduces symptoms of upset stomach, reduces osteoarthritis pain, possible relief of skin cancer.

Acai juice. High in antioxidants.

Quinoa. High in protein, all nine essential amino acids, use it to replace rice.

Chia seeds. A regular of mine. The most essential fatty acids of any known plant. High in antioxidants, iron, magnesium, calcium, potassium, high in fiber.

Almonds. Another daily snack. The most nutritionally dense nut, high in fiber, potassium, calcium, vitamin E, magnesium and iron.

Pumpkin seeds. Another daily. High in antioxidants, fiber, protein, zinc, vitamin K, phosphorus, manganese, calcium, iron, fatty acids, potassium, vitamin B2, reduces chances of stomach, breast, lung and colon cancer, improves prostrate and bladder health, high in magnesium which is important for controlling blood pressure and reducing heart disease risk, improves heart health, sperm quality, sleep.

Lemon. Another regular. High in antioxidants, cancer fighting, helps prevent diabetes, high blood pressure, fever, indigestion, improves skin, hair, teeth, contains vitamins C, B6, A, E, folate, niacin and more, drinking lemon juice with luke warm water and honey promotes weight loss.

Cayenne Pepper. A great body cleanser, stimulates circulation and neutralizes acidity, anti-irritant, clears congestion, anti-fungal, joint pain relief, detoxifies the body, great with honey and lemon with a teaspoon of lemon in the morning, anti-bacterial, supports weight-loss, helps prevent cancer, high in antioxidants.

Apple cider vinegar. Natural cleanser and alkanizer of body. Improves blood sugar levels, aids natural weight loss. Reduces inflammation. Take a table spoon with a mug fo warm water.

Ajwa dates and ajwa seed powder. Highly effective for blocked arteries, helps prevent cancer, provides energy, promotes weight loss, high in antioxidants.

There are numerous more 'superfoods', find which ones suit you, ones which your physiology requires, that suit your taste, or just create your own mix, just be consistent, small portions, regularly for the long-term.

I have my own concoctions I do regularly. When I used to box, my diet would be a low carbohydrate and high protein one, and in the morning I would have water, lemon and a teaspoon of cayenne pepper.

If you are a male, food containing zinc and magnesium is beneficial for sperm quality and testosterone production.

My current favorite concoction is green tea, with honey, ajwa seed powder and fresh ginger.

I put chia seeds in whatever I cook, i.e. an omelet. Pumpkin seeds I have daily with almonds, a handful a day.

According to the Harvard School of Public Health, how you 'design' your dinner plate, can help your nutritional intake. Half of your plate should consist of fruit and vegetables, aim for color and variety, potatoes don't count because of their effect on blood sugar.

One quarter of your plate should be wholegrains. Quinoa, oats, brown rice, or whole wheat pasta.

One quarter of your plate should be protein. Such as fish and chicken. Limit your red meat intake.

Choose healthy vegetable oils like olive oil, sunflower, peanut.

Drink water, coffee or tea. No fizzy drinks, limit juice to one glass per day, limit milk and dairy to one serving per day. A note here, avoid drinking before your meal, it fills the stomach before you can finish your meal. My normal routine now is, carbonated water, to get that fizzy drink feeling, half way through my meal I would have half a glass, then finish the other half at the end of my meal. Carbonated water on its own or with a diluted fruit juice is a 'healthier' alternative to fizzy drinks. I would then have a probiotic yoghurt as a desert, followed by decaffeinated green tea. Place a cardamom pod in the mug to alter the taste of green tea which can be bitter.

Remember, focus on *quality* not just quantity, the type of carbohydrate etc. The Healthy Eating Plate guidelines according to the Harvard School of Public Health contribute to the reduction in risk of developing heart disease and premature death.

Write down your shopping list, correlate it to what is in this chapter, put a tick against what is okay, put a cross against what is not okay, write next to it the foods you can replace it with. Use this as your new shopping list now, try new recipes. If you must use unhealthy refined carbohydrates, sugary drinks etc. do so sparingly. Treat yourself once a week. Set goals and targets, if you run a certain number of miles or do some other physical activity, allow yourself a treat – once! If you attend (if needed) a therapeutic session for your mental health, treat yourself, if you diet all week, treat yourself on the weekend. If you want to be serious, and make serious improvements, that are noticeable within two weeks, train like a hurricane with no treats and no breaks! If you find adapting and making changes too difficult, remember the philosophy of The Monk Life; small, consistent changes over the long term. What you put into your body, is what you will get out. Which brings me to *supplements*.

Supplements offer us an alternative to provide us with the nutrients we require. According to the Harvard Medical School, most studies conducted on supplements were *observational* trials, meaning they weren't in a controlled setting, nor tested against a 'placebo'. When the rigorous evidence is available from randomized *controlled* trials, they are often at odds with the findings of the observational trials.

Some supplements proved to be not only ineffective but also risky. Vitamin E, which was initially thought to protect the heart, was later discovered to increase the risk for bleeding strokes. Folic acid and other B vitamins were once believed to prevent heart disease and strokes, until later studies not only didn't confirm that benefit but actually raised concerns that high doses of these nutrients might increase cancer risk.

For nutrients, I would personally stick to food, build a vast supply of superfoods at home, and only take supplements if advised by a physician. I have tried many supplements over the years - vitamins, amino acids and countless more. It is all trial and error, you might find that one may work for you. However, I will list what I have tried that has worked for me, a 40 year old male.

The most common natural supplement I can speak of its effectiveness is ZMA, which contains zinc, magnesium, calcium and vitamin B6, taken before bed it aids recovery, improves sleep and elevates testosterone levels.
Another, is Icariin extract, a natural herbal supplement which enhances testosterone levels. However these have varied effects, I would limit these to one or two periods a year, or when you feel that you need it, get yourself checked with the doctor to see if you need to elevate your levels. It's possible, you do not and sometimes these supplements can give you unwanted side effects such as mood swings. Nevertheless, enhancing testosterone levels is imperative for males over thirty. I find a combo of supplements works well, however I normally refrain from taking more than one or two types at any one time. If you take multiple supplements together, you will never know which one is working for you.

Fish oil is a very good daily supplement.
Tongkat Ali is another recommended natural herbal supplement, probably the 1:200 extract or 1:50 in powdered form, direct from Pasak Bumi in Indonesia. However, I would recommend trial and error, small doses, as this can work as much as it can give you an unwanted mood swing. I would add the powdered form to my coffee or tea in the morning, great before a run. If supplements have side effects, take them at bedtime, if you can sleep on them,

taking them at bedtime means you will sleep through the side effects, as well as being the best time to take hormone enhancing supplements. This is because when you sleep, your body releases testosterone and growth hormone. Your job is to create the optimal conditions for your body to do this, including going to sleep for your peak period.

We never know what's going in a herbal pill, this is an unregulated market, check your sources, be wary, the body is *thy* temple, fifty pounds a month on your favorite magic pill could pay for a bottle of ZMA, and a few months' supply of goji berries, pumpkin seeds, almonds, etc. I would opt for the latter, as that is where I have seen the best results, *naturally.*

If you combine eating well with chapter ones regime of deadlifts, squats etc., you will see elevated levels of the right hormones in your body, including testosterone and growth hormone.
We are talking life changes here, small changes to benefit you, your health, I can relate to athletes, I can relate to the overweight, I can relate to those with bouts of depression, or neglected, it all comes down to *your* 'will'.
Get a whiteboard, write down your goals, small, attainable goals that can be achieved in a day, a week. Keep that whiteboard in front of you, see it, visualize it, when you sleep, when you wake up, every time you walk into your room. For example:
First goal, 'Stop buying coke',
Second goal, 'replace with water/carbonated water',
Third goal, 'jog two miles',
Fourth goal, 'ring different counsellors for an informal chat',
Fifth goal, 'eat portion of goji berries a day'.
These are all simplistic, attainable goal that you can alter to suit your desires. You can change jog to brisk walk, or spin

class. Goji to pumpkin seeds, or to lemon, water, cayenne mix (if you're brave – benefit far outweighs the displeasure). Every time you complete a goal, cross it out, don't wipe it off, wait until you complete all five, then take a photo of it as evidence, to remind yourself what you are capable of, then write down five more small, attainable goals. Step by step, you will get there.

Central Power is not a magic wand, I wish it was, but it does help a great deal. The foundation techniques in the first chapter will improve your health and fitness, combine it with the next three chapters, and you have The Monk Life.

'Knowing is not enough, we must apply. Willing is not enough, we must do'.
-*Bruce Lee.*

EPILOGUE

These ancient techniques, are like fine tuning your engine, your body, to achieve what it is truly capable of, of *more*. More and more studies are being done to prove the notion that we can conjure up more abilities from within us. This book is designed to do that, to give you the ability to be stronger, better, more robust, upright, sturdy, focused and disciplined.

I hope I have assisted you in some way, I hope after hours, weeks, months of practice you notice the difference. I am available for comment, advice, tips, on social media. I am also available for one to one or group lessons, contact me to learn more. If you want to learn at the heart, in Indonesia, I can refer you to my colleagues whom are excellent in this field.

Remember The Monk Life philosophy, small, consistent steps, towards your goals, for the long term. If you are in competition, remember there is a fine line between victory and defeat, only those who train, harder, longer, with more *intellect* applied than their opponents, will succeed.

I wish you well, my aim with this book is to serve you, I hope it serves you well.

Your friend,

Ali 'Sugar Ray'.

REFERENCES

Information has been taken from the following sources, with credit and thanks to:

The National Centre for Biotechnology Information
https://www.ncbi.nlm.nih.gov/pmc/articles/PMC1402378/
https://www.ncbi.nlm.nih.gov/pubmed/21291246
https://www.ncbi.nlm.nih.gov/pmc/articles/PMC3057175/
https://www.ncbi.nlm.nih.gov/pubmedhealth/PMH0027030/
https://www.ncbi.nlm.nih.gov/pubmed/28954895
Science Daily
https://www.sciencedaily.com/releases/2017/11/1711221035
55.htm
https://www.sciencedaily.com/releases/2017/09/1709071124
08.htm
BMJ Postgraduate Medical Journals
http://pmj.bmj.com/content/90/1059/26
American Osteopathic Association
http://www.osteopathic.org/osteopathic-health/about-your-
health/health-conditions-library/general-
health/Pages/yoga.aspx
Yoga Journal
https://www.yogajournal.com/poses/cobra-pose
Arogya Yoga School
https://arogyayogaschool.com/blog/10-health-benefits-of-
cobra-pose-bhujangasana/
The Independent
http://www.independent.co.uk/news/uk/home-news/self-
harm-teenage-girls-increase-three-years-up-68-per-cent-
research-a8008711.html

http://www.independent.co.uk/news/uk/home-news/leading-mental-health-bodies-warn-government-the-crisis-is-here-a8035776.html
Health.com
http://www.health.com/depression/8-million-americans-psychological-distress
MIND, for better mental health
https://www.mind.org.uk/information-support/drugs-and-treatments/mindfulness/mindfulness-courses/#.WiWSjLacY0q
https://www.mind.org.uk/information-support/types-of-mental-health-problems/mental-health-problems-introduction/treatment-options/#.WiWSobacY0q
Hypnotherapy Directory
http://www.hypnotherapy-directory.org.uk/content/industryfaqs.html
http://www.hypnotherapy-directory.org.uk/approach/suggestion-hypnotherapy.html
Psychology Today
https://www.psychologytoday.com/blog/what-mentally-strong-people-dont-do/201611/7-ways-use-your-mind-strengthen-and-heal-your-body
NHS Medical Research Council
https://www.mrc.ac.uk/documents/pdf/review-of-nutrition-and-human-health/
British Nutrition Foundation
https://www.nutrition.org.uk/healthyliving/basics/exploring-nutrients.html?limit=1&start=1
Harvard School of Public Health
https://www.hsph.harvard.edu/nutritionsource/best-diet-quality-counts/
https://www.hsph.harvard.edu/nutritionsource/healthy-eating-plate/

https://www.health.harvard.edu/staying-healthy/dietary-supplements-do-they-help-or-hurt

GuideDoc.com

http://guidedoc.com/best-superfoods-list

Healthline.com

https://www.healthline.com/nutrition/11-benefits-of-pumpkin-seeds

azcentral

https://healthyliving.azcentral.com/supposed-lay-flat-sit-ups-19467.html

Forbes

https://www.forbes.com/sites/daviddisalvo/2017/11/29/how-breathing-calms-your-brain-and-other-science-based-benefits-of-controlled-breathing/#3e71b3e52221

Science

http://science.sciencemag.org/content/355/6332/1411/tab-figures-data

Hypertension

http://hyper.ahajournals.org/content/46/4/714.short

The Journal of Neuroscience

http://www.jneurosci.org/content/36/49/12448

PLOS ONE

http://journals.plos.org/plosone/article?id=10.1371/journal.pone.0062817

The Bruce Lee Family Company

https://www.brucelee.com/family-company

Science Alert

http://www.sciencealert.com/extreme-diet-reverse-type-2-diabetes-up-to-86-patients-remission-weight

The Lancet

http://www.thelancet.com/journals/lancet/article/PIIS0140-6736%2817%2933102-1/fulltext?elsca1=tlpr

Muhammad Ali

https://muhammadali.com

ACKNOWLEDGEMENTS

I would like to acknowledge, in no order of preference:

My teacher in Indonesia, Mr Rahmatan aka 'Bang Ote'
Everyone who trained with me in Indonesia, including my
deceased friend Andrey Chilling (may God bless his soul)
who introduced me to Bang Ote and to Daniel Lee who
introduced me to Andrey, Ivanka Slank and the band SLANK
for always having my back in Jakarta, Masha Sutardjo, Geri
Xakala, Rulionzo, Quint, the original crew who trained with
me
Everyone from Cawang, Jakarta
'Bruce Lee', my original inspiration
Muhammad Ali, my original inspiration
Sugar Ray Robinson, Joe Louis, Rocky Marciano
Other boxers and fighters who have inspired me, Prince
Naseem Hamed, Roberto Duran, Manny Pacquiao, Floyd
Mayweather, Sugar Ray Leonard, Mike Tyson, Reggie
Johnson, Julio Cesar Chavez, Salvador Sanchez, GGG, Canelo
and so on, too many to mention
Everyone who laces up the gloves
Everyone in combat sports
Every Paralympian that ever existed
Every Olympian that ever existed
Every *athlete*
Every coach & trainer
Every disabled person
Everyone inflicted by disease or injury
Everyone suffering with their own battles be it mental
health, overweight or something else
Every elderly person
Everyone serving the community in their own form

Tyson Fury for overcoming his health issues
Anthony Joshua
Billy Joe Saunders for showing how travelers fight
Everyone I boxed with over the years including all the gyms
in Bradford, Round One, K.O gym and all the boys, Fiz and
all my friends from Bradford, Nadeem Siddique and his crew,
for believing in me, Nettles Nasser for finding me on
Myspace in 2007 and inviting me to train with the U.S
Contender Team in Newcastle, three time World Champ
'Sweet' Reggie Johnson for his friendship with me over my
years in boxing, Spencer Fearon for believing in me and his
advice when I moved to London, 'Uncle', Mustapha and all
the boys I boxed with in London, including Darren Hamilton
who sparred with me, so I can say I sparred with a
welterweight British Champ, Shabba Shafiq from
Sw33tscience Inc, Pak Bayu & Brother Am for having my
back in Bali over the years. Nick for holding the Iron plate,
my boys in London Hissan and Shaz
Everyone who supported me over the years
My family, friends, all who knew that this book was coming
Ferheen Baig (PhD Cardiovascular Research Kings College
London)
Indonesia – I *salute* you
Cover by @yonatanugerah
Matthew Raza

ABOUT THE AUTHOR

His other book is The Pilgrim, a Story & Guide to Hajj and Umrah for Muslims and non-Muslims alike.

Printed in Great Britain
by Amazon

82521142R00058